HOSPITAL MANAGEMENT

Management Executives Handbook–Series 009

HOSPITAL MANAGEMENT

SAVITA SHARMA • K'CHERRY

Commonwealth

in association with

NATIONAL CENTRE FOR HEALTH MANAGEMENT

Hospital Management

Edition : **2027**

ISBN 81-7169-390-3

Published by :
COMMONWEALTH PUBLISHERS (P) LTD.
4831/24, Govind Lane,
Ansari Road, Darya Ganj,
New Delhi - 110002
Ph. : 23272541, 23242541
e-mail : commonwealthpublishers2016@gmail.com

Distributed by :
ARJUN PUBLISHING HOUSE
4831/24, Govind Lane,
Ansari Road, Darya Ganj,
New Delhi - 110002
Ph. : 23272541, 23242541
e-mail : arjunbooks2001@gmail.com

Laser Typesetting by :
Dimple Computers
Delhi

Printed at :
Milan Enterprises
Delhi

Preface

We believe various professionals will be interested in the material this book presents. Students enrolled in health programs in health services administration will find this a useful source. It can serves as a reference text for instructor, lecture and/or class discussion. Finally, we anticipate that busy managers employed by hospitals and other health services institutions will find this book a practical tool.

May be thirty or forty years ago the total body of literature on hospital administration was fully within a singly individual's capacity to review, and even perhaps to own. Today, that body reflects an explosive and relentless expansion similar in magnitude to that which began among the professional medical specialities much earlier. If one thing becomes necessary in the face of this avalanche of material—both good and bad-it is the exercise of selectivity.

Those of us engaged in management of modern health care institutions owe out compliments. This book instructs, enlightens, and provokes. It will prove inspiring to some, and useful to all.

Editors

Contents

1 The Hospital as an Organisation

Persons representing a variety of disciplines have turned their attention to health care. Operations researchers, engineers, accountants, attorneys, political scientists, and politicians are participating in health care administration. Hospital are the major recipient of this increased attention. In addition to being highly visible, bricks-and-mortar organizations, hospitals are suggested as the focal point of health care services has also focused on hospitals.

For hospitals and their personnel, from governing authority on down, this is future shock. Hospitals are faced with new environments and confronted with new rules. Many of the old assumptions regarding hospitals and their philosophies are being challenged. Those in leadership positions, both within and outside the health care field, have asserted that there is a health care crisis. Although it is a crisis with many facets, it is not a crisis to cause the system to collapse or disintegrate. Questions are raised about the costs and the efficacy of medical care, the desirability of receiving it, the fallibility of the physician, and the ability of the health care system to save people from imprudent lifestyles, unhealthy environment, and individual genetic makeup. Best stated, it is a crisis of confidence.

Complexity of hospitals

The hospitals has been and continues to be one of the most complex organizations in existence. This complexity requires organizational arrangements which have been termed by some authors as prototypical, e.g., task teams composed of a wide variety of skilled professionals are commonplace in hospitals. Some theorists who have conducted studies about hospitals are surprised that such institutions functions at all.

The complexity of the modern hospital results from a number of attributes:

1. *Within the institution, there is a wide diversity of objectives and goals for different personnel and subsystems.* Various segments of the hospital will be responsible for, or involved in, patient care, education, research, hotel-type accommodations and problems, and carrying out complex and sophisticated medical and surgical procedures. These various activities are sometimes contradictory and often in conflict.

2. *The diversity of personnel ranges from the most highly skilled and educated physicians and administrators to unskilled and uneducated employees.* Enabling them to work together is a major responsibility of the hospital manager.

3. *The hospital is in continuous operation.* This requires high standby costs and involves substantial personnel and scheduling problems.
4. *In many areas of hospital operations there are dual lines of authority.* Administrators are responsible for solving a wide variety of management problems, and physicians are responsible for patient care, education, and research. Often these two seemingly distinct areas of activity overlap, and, in fact, some employees may have two or more persons to whom they are responsible.
5. *Hospitals deal with problems of life and death.* This puts a special psychological and physical stress on personnel at all levels of the organization—it is not the usual service organization. Often the setting and results case consumers to be hypercritical.
6. *There is a problem in measuring the major product.* The patient care rendered in the hospital has eluded precise measurement. Although there has been some progress in determining the quality of care, many questions remain unanswered and substantial disagreement exists among the experts as to how and what should be measured.

These attributes are unlikely to change. In fact, increasingly the technology used by hospitals is more expensive and complicated; therefore, managing the institution is likely to become more difficult.

Historical development of hospitals

Historically, the earliest evidence of institutionalized care for the ill can be found about 1200 B.C. in Greek temples. Hippocrates, the most prominent Greek physician, was instrumental in separating medicine from religion and philosophy. He is credited with addressing medicine from a rational standpoint and the foundations of modern medicine are built upon his work. Medical training gained importance in this era, as did recognition of environmental influences on health and disease. Religion, however, undoubtedly continued to play a fundamental role in the development of hospitals.

Greek medicine reached its zenith during the Golden Age of Greece, about 400 B.C., when the temples of Aseculapius emerged. Considered among the earliest hospitals in Greek and Roman civilizations, the temples were used both as houses of worship and as shelters for the diseased. The patients were often ambulatory. The care in Aesculapia was non-brutal, emphasizing patient exposure to the open air and sunshine as well as a regimen of rest, relaxation, baths, exercise, and proper diet. Such temples were similar in nature to modern day spas—the individual and his body were given the support for recuperation and restoration to health. Limited medication was prescribed to patients at the Aesculapia; the records show that many did regain their health as a result of these simple regimens.

The first hospitals evidencing modern features were found in ancient Egypt and India. In Egypt, at approximately 600 B.C., medical care was often rendered in healing temples. Egyptian priest-physicians were among the first to prescribe practical drugs, and they performed limited surgery and set fractures. Between 273-232 B.C. hospitals called Cikista were built in India. Hindu physicians were adept surgeons and medications were administered. Such institutions were noted for their high state of cleanliness and sanitation. Patients remained overnight and were carded for by attendants.

Hospitals and early christianity

The Christian era stressed humanitarianism. During that period ecclesiastic hostels were built adjacent to churches so that priests could conveniently care for and offer solace to patients. By the year 500 A.D., almost every city throughout the old Roman empire had established church-related hospitals. Religious beliefs superseded scientific, Hippocratic knowledge in treatment of patients. Christianity prevailed in the provision of medical care, emphasizing above all else the importance of compassion and care for each patient, often at the expense of scientific knowledge.

After the fall of Rome, and especially during the Middle Ages, hospitals were marked by increasingly strong religious influence. Medical advances used in India, Egypt, and the Roman empire were lost as these civilizations disintegrated During the Middle Ages, a very bleak period for hospitals, medical knowledge which had been developed went unused, primarily because of social and religious pressures. Renewed emphasis on supernatural influences in health and disease occurred as the Christian church gained a prominent role in dictating the processes of medical treatment.

The middle East did not have the decline in the quality of medicine which occurred in western Europe during the Middle Ages. Mohammedan physicians were acquainted with use of inhalation anesthesia and they originated the use of a vast number of new drugs. Moslem countries had asylums for the mentally ill a thousand years before such institutions appeared in Europe. Built in Cairo in the 13th century, Al-Mansur Hospital was equipped with separate wards for more serious diseases, had outpatient clinics, and operated homes for the convalescent.

The renaissance

The value of scientific medical knowledge was not rediscovered until the Renaissance, beginning in the 14th century. Ironically though Christianity was a major inhibiting force in the use of such medical knowledge, much of it was recorded in books prepared and preserved by monasteries during the Middle Ages. As the writings of early Greeks were revived, 16th century scholars applied their knowledge in the development of new scientific theories. This rebirth of interest in scientific medicine encouraged physicians to attempt procedures which exceeded their knowledge of science and their ability to prevent or understand the consequences of their actions. The hospital's reputation was not enhanced by these increasingly daring surgeons. During the late 18th and early 19th centuries, wound infection was ubiquitous and puss drainage was considered a sign of healing. Brutal medical treatment such as bleeding, purging, violent emetics, and cathartics were commonly used. A good surgeon was one who could operate quickly—the lack of anesthesia made the patient's pain unbearable and he was rather difficult to control.

The hospital had shifted from religious orientation to medical orientation. The Renaissance succeeded in substantially separating science from religion, establishing clearly the scientific approach to medical matters. Although religious conflicts were to emerge occasionally, scientific inquiry finally became the dominant influence in medical care delivery.

The oldest existing hospital in western Europe is the Hotel-Dieu, Paris, France, founded in A.D. 550 and rebuilt in the 13th century. Malcolm T. MacEachern, hospital historian, writer, an theorist, describes it as a hospital not unlike today's facility. In its construction the importance of separating individuals in different disease states and various stages of recovery was emphasized and the hospital was divided into wards. For instance, there were sections for convalescent and maternity patients. Departments with specialized functions were directed/ by a department head, and others were assigned to specialty tasks such as food, drugs, laundry, and dressings. A kind of governing authority, the board of provisors, inspected the institution twice a year.

Period of growth (1860-1920)

The first hospital in the United States, the Pennsylvania Hospital, was founded in 1751. In 1798 Congress passed legislation establishing the Marine Hospital Service for merchant seamen. However, in the United States, 1860 to 1920 was the period of explosive hospital growth. Hospitals increased from several hundred in the 1870s to a peak of 7,370 in 1924. During these years medicine evolved from an age of ignorance to an age of basic technology and science. Advances during this period laid the foundation for 20th century medicine and the modern hospital. The discovery of anesthesia in the late 1840s was the first of many events which led to changes in medical philosophy and treatment modes. The homeopaths and eclectic medical sects reached a peak of influence, but declined as allopathic medicine matured after the turn of the century. The heroic and vigorous therapy treatment modes gave way to those based on scientific knowledge. Use of antiseptic surgery in the 1860s yielded to aseptic surgery based on the germ theory of disease after the bacteriologists discovered the link between micro-organisms and disease. Koch's study of anthrax and tuberculosis, and Pasteur's work with rabies and cholera in the 1880s were part of these break-throughs.

Diagnostic techniques also contributed to the emerging role of the hospital. Roentgen's discovery of the X-ray in 1895, blood typing in 1990 development of the electrocardiograph in 1902 , and the Curies, experimentation with radium were only a few of the era's scientific advances.

These developments permitted surgeons to increase their intervention in disease processes and to do so with decreasing mortality and greater efficacy. A place for the focus of this technology had to be found. Hospitals, already established, offered surgeons a physical facility, equipment, personnel and perhaps most importantly, an organizational framework within which modern surgery could be performed. Primarily, the development of the 20th century hospital is a history of the growth of efficacious surgery.

Also during this period medical education evolved from a state of "nonenlightenment" to one which bogan to utilizc the growing scientific base. Before 1990 most medical schools were proprietary. Their entrance requirements were minimal and exit requirements were not much higher. Most did not have laboratory facilities or clinical training for their students. In 1893 the Johns Hopkins medical school was formed. Modeled after German universities, it soon became the premier American institution for medical education. It was the first to require an undergraduate degree as part of its admission requirements, and the first to have four years of study, as compared with two years in most of the other 131 schools.

In 1910, Abraham Flexner was commissioned

by the Carnegie Foundation to evaluate all medical schools in the United States and Canada. Some major deficiencies reported were: low or nonexistent admission standards; poor facilities; inadequate staff; and lack of basic science and clinical instruction. The issuance of the Flexner report was a turning point in medical education, and it was to have a major impact on hospitals.

Concurrent developments helped to shape the modern hospital's role; emergence of nursing as a profession, and changes in society's attitudes toward hospitals. Preceding the Crimean War, nursing was often performed by religious orders. Sectarian nursing had low status and standards, and attracted persons who sometimes abused and robbed their patients. However, the period 1860-1920 witnessed advances in nursing, expansion of the nurse's role in health care delivery, and establishment of professional schools of nursing. Florence Nightingale, a pioneer in English nursing, and Dorothea Dix, a pioneer in American nursing, were instrumental in fostering these changes. The first three schools of nursing in the United States were established in 1873. In 1890 there were 35 schools of nursing; by 1910 there were 1,129. The role of these new professionals began evolving to a partnership with physicians in the delivery of health care.

The change in society's attitude toward the role of hospitals in delivering health care did not occur quickly. Crowded and unsanitary conditions, high mortality rates, and meager medical care deterred people from entering hospitals voluntarily. These conditions and attitudes were changing; the industrialization of the United States during the 1860-1920 period and the urbanization of our society assisted the growth of hospitals. As society became more urbanized sanitation worsened, and slum conditions and the spread of diseases became more prevalent. In many instances hospitals became the place for care of those individuals migrating to the cities. Finally, a shift in attitude occurred; the hospital was seen less as a charitable institution and it was respectable for a paying patient to be admitted. The 1947 Commission on Hospital Care indicated that the "lack of public interest, because of ignorance and prejudice, resulted in slow hospital growth and a low quality of service during early periods. Once prejudice was eliminated then illness rather than economic status was recognized as the basis for hospital admission. The pay-patient system assisted the expansion of hospitals by disassociating "Hospital" from the connotation of charity.

Consolidation (1920-1950)

By 1920 the foundation had been laid. In the following thirty years refinements were made and consolidation occurred. In 1924 there were 7,370 hospitals in the United States, the highest number ever. By 1950 there were 6,788 hospitals; however, the total number of beds increased from 813,000 in 1924 to 1,456, 000. At the end of the period more beds were located in fewer facilities and the quality of care provided improved dramatically. Two significant events which had a major impact on hospitals during this period were accreditation and the beginning of private health insurance.

In 1913, the American College of Surgeons was formed. Criteria for physicians seeking fellowship included submission of one hundred case histories of patients on whom the surgeon had operated. Discovering that many could not do so because hospitals had inadequate patient records, the College outlined a set of requirements including: medical staff, patient records, and diagnostic and therapeutic equipment requirements. These had to be met before a hospital was placed on its approved list. This process was carried out by the college until 1951 when its activities were transferred to the Joint Commission on Accreditation Hospitals.

The impact of approval by the American College of Surgeons was to force the closing of many substandard hospitals. In addition, the College's standards hastened acquisition and use of therapeutic and diagnostic equipment in hospital and the establishment of laboratories. Consequently, it was an important force in reshaping the hospital, altering its role in developing as the major element in the delivery of health care.

The second major event affecting hospitals in this period was the emergence of private hospitalization insurance plans. One of the earliest, the between the Baylor University Hospital and 1500 local teachers, was signed in 1929. For a fixed fee the hospital agreed to provide, if necessary, up to 21 days of hospitalization to each subscriber. By the mid 1940s there were 87 private hospitalization plans covering over 20 million people. The effect was substantial. First, they kept a number of hospitals from going bankrupt during the depression. Second, they enabled enrollees to prevent the financial disaster of a major illness by spreading risk over a larger enrolled population. Third, they permitted the fee-for-service health care delivery system to become further entrenched. Finally, they helped consolidated hospitals as the major institution in the health care delivery system.

Unlike its European contemporaries, the American hospital system was largely developed and built without government involvement. The vast general acute hospital network which emerged in the United States from 1900 through the end of World War II was predominantly the product of voluntary initiative on the part of the American people and of certain religious groups. Government participation in health care at the federal level was limited to special groups: servicemen, veterans, American Indians, and merchant mariners: and psychiatric hospitals at the state level. A large number of city and country government hospitals were built.

Hospital organization

Voluntary not-for-profit hospitals evolved some unique aspects. The most important of these was the sharing of power in a triad, which includes the governing authority, and chief executive officer and medical staff. Theoretically, this arrangement permits a sharing of power among the three participants, but can best be characterized as-an accommodation. The triad results from: the independent contractor status of staff physicians who care for their patients in the hospital and the need for governing authorities to delegate responsibility for day to-day operation of the facility to an administrator. Despite its many shortcomings and the increasing number of attacks on its efficiency and desirability, the triad has continued to be the dominant form of organization for voluntary, non-for-profit hospitals.

New models

Recently, a new title has been proposed for the largest category of hospitals. It is suggested that "public general" hospital is a more meaningful generic grouping for all hospitals which offer a broad range of medical and surgical services to the public at large. This title includes hospitals of all types of ownership which serve more than a select group of beneficiaries or specific disease entities and recognizes the quasipublic utility status which hospitals have.

A new organizational model proposed for voluntary not-for-profit hospitals is the corporate structure. In this form the governing authority delegates power to a chief executive officer who is responsible for all activities within the facility, including medical care. While this may be desirable from an administrative standpoint, it ignores the power and influence of medical staffs generally, and is likely to gain acceptance slowly, if at all.

Closer links between the chief executive officer and the governing authority may tend to minimize the CEO's independence. However, only in hospitals where physicians are employed has there been established a greater degree of line authority over physicians—at least over the administrative aspects of hospital medical practice. By the very nature of the physician's education and professional activity, however, functional independence is a necessary and desirable element. In investor-owned, not-for-profit, and other community hospitals, medical staffs retain a high degree of independence and in most situations hospitals have relied on moral suasion to gain physical cooperation. Increasingly, however, this may not be adequate. The courts have declared that despite the lack of an employment relationship, the hospital, through its governing authority, is accountable for the medical practice rendered. The inevitable result of this will be increased control of what physicians do and a greater willingness to use sanctions such as limitation or suspension of hospital privileges. Attenuating or removing privileges is the most director control point which hospital privilege. Attenuating or removing privileges is the most direct control point which hospitals have over physicians; however, this happens only rarely.

The governing authority

As the result of diverse pressures the hospital

board of trustees or as it is increasingly called, the governing authority, has come under close scrutiny. These pressure include community interest, governmental regulation, third party pay or involvement, and malpractice decisions. Boards are often asked pointed questions about community responsibility and involvement. Court decisions on malpractice have sharpened the accountability of governing authorities for medical staff activities. Increasing economic difficulties have made a through understanding of financial matters imperative. To remedy these problems, various proposal have been made to increase competence of governing authority members, especially in technical areas. These proposals include seminars, continuing education, and outside resources such as consultants.

Based on previous experience, these suggestions for developing internal competence of a voluntary board must be questioned. To do so in no way belittles or besmirches the conscientious efforts of thousands of participants nation wide. The demands being placed on them have changed dramatically, primarily because the hospital's environment is so different.

Trustees of voluntary hospital governing authorities have traditionally come from the educated and upper socioeconomic groups. Board membership for the hospital chief executive officer and/or hospital physician was roundly debated for many years. Its undesirability is infrequently mentioned today and increasing numbers of hospitals include both.

The increasing accountability of governing authority members is likely to result in a natural selection process. The ramifications of membership will cull those individuals who have neither the time nor the expertise to be truly effective. Nonchalant of superficial involvement is likely to become a thing of the past. It is doubtful that even the most effective education program can do more than partially offset the chronic shortage of time which most members experience. It has been suggested that the hospital administrative staff should provide the expertise to assist governing authority members. Consultants have also been used as means to offset this deficit. Of the two, more highly qualified administrative staff is probably a better solution. However, neither approach is adequate. Policy decisions of acceptable qualify by the governing authority can only result when the membership has virtually as much expertise as do CEOs and their staffs or consultants especially in terms to the external forces. One is led, therefore, to conclusion that evolution will be toward paid governing authority numbers who devote a specific amount of time to governance of a facility and are paid for that time-a pattern long since adopted by business boards.

For those governing authority members who are defined as trustees there are additional burdens of serving. In the eyes of the law, trustees are similar to fiduciaries. They are held to a very high standard of conduct. They are charged with safeguarding the assets of the organization, protecting the patient from harm, and not getting any secret personal gain from their relationship. Conflict of interest—or more precisely stated, differing interests-on the parts of trustees has increasingly been the subject of journalistic and legal inquiries. Recent court decisions have identified nonfeasance as an important a shortcoming as malfeasance. This increasing emphasis on ethical conduct for governing authority members will make even honest candidates less likely to want to serve.

The administrator

MacEachern identified Florence Nightingale, an Englishwoman, as the first hospital administrator. Since Nightingale did her work during the mid-19th century, his conclusion makes emergence of the hospital executive a relatively recent phenomenon. Hospital administration was identified as having a distinct body of knowledge when the University of Chicago established the first U.S graduate program in hospital administration 1934. The number of programmes increased slowly during the years that followed, until the mid-1960s when a period of rapid growth occurred. In 1976 there were 35 graduate education programs accredited the Accrediting Commission on Education for Health Services Administration. There are numerous graduate and undergraduate programs not accredited, but the growth of undergraduate education has been most explosive -it is estimated there are well over 100 nation wide.

Hospital managers are educated in a variety

of institutional setting: schools of business, public health, economics, and medicine. Similarly the content within these setting is different, but one requirement for accreditation is that certain types of subject matter be taught. This is consistent with the development of a distinct body of knowledge in the field—albeit eclectic. The Master's degree is usually awarded after two years of study, divided into didactic and residency portions of varying lengths. Most programs contend they are educating generalist managers for top leadership positions.

Among hospital managers there is a continuing discourse about whether the field of hospital administration has achieved professional stature. There is little doubt that it has been professionalized through use of education, income, titles, and other accouterments of office. Furthermore, hospital personnel-including physicians-and the public generally recognize the role and importance of hospital managers. However, hospital managers have not joined the ranks of the historic learned professions, e.g., law, medicine, and the clergy. In addition, there continues to be evidence that many physicians do not consider administrators to be their peers.

As the hospital administrator became a usual entity in the hospital hierarchy a primary task was to implement policy developed by the governing authority. Depending on the relative strengths and weaknesses of the board vis-a-vis the administrator, the scopes of their roles have been quite varIed. Within the past ten years, however, the importance of external forces on hospitals has grown dramatically. We have reached the point where hospitals are so influenced by external forces, that the two individuals are commonly responsible for hospital activities. One is charged with managing the internal functioning of the facility: the second, usually the superior, interacts in and evaluates the external environment of the hospital and makes this knowledge and information available to the governing authority and the internal management. Regardless of the specific approach used, there is no doubt that the hospital executive will have to be increasingly well-educated and sophisticated to function effectively in the health care environment: above all, leadership and management skills are required.

The medical staff

The medical staff is an indispensible element of hospital operation Society has recognized the physician as having unique knowledge and ability in dealing with the ill. Through the licensing process it verifies that this individual has, in fact, achieved basic abilities. By virtue of the license, then, the physician is permitted to exercise a number of powers which are not given to others, e.g., control of prescription drugs. This power is found in hospitals- the whole treatment of hospital in and out-patients is dependent on the physician personally carrying out medical treatment and/or directing and supervising others in performing certain tasks. This importance, in addition to professional independence and social status, has necessitated a relationship in the hospital hierarchy in which physician have substantial power. This unique relationship has added immensely to the complexity of hospital management and organization.

The hospital-based specialists, e.g., anesthesiologists and pathologists, are often employees; increasingly full-time chiefs-of-staff and chiefs-of-service are being hired. This has occurred because proper management by physicians of medical activities can no longer be done on a part-time or voluntary basis. This change is not only consistent with good management practice, but is necessitated by increasing emphasis on scrutinizing hospitals and holding them accountable for the quality of medical care.

Often, persons unfamiliar with the American hospital system and hospital organization are surprised to learn that the physicians pay nothing for the privilege of treating patients in the facility. At the time when hospitals had charity wards, and physicians contributed their time and effort to treating those patients, there was a true exchange between the facility and the physician. The physician assisted the hospital in meeting a prime social responsibility-caring for indigent patients. At present there are few patients for whom no payment is received by either hospital or physician. The question of what it is that the physician contributes to the hospital has been asked in some quarters. Is it a symbiotic relationship from which society benefits, and is this fact alone adequate? Or does the hospital provide an indispensible workshop, which, if not provided by the hospital, would have to be furnished by the physician? Neither can function without the other, yet the relationship probably more beneficial to the physician than it is to the facility.

The long-term trend will likely result in greater control by hospitals over physicians. Increased demands for accountability from government, consumer, and third-party payor will bring this about. It may well be that the end result in hospital-based specialists-specialist physician attached to hospital without office practices.

The hospital is today and likely will remain one of the most complex and fascinating organizational entities in existence. Hospital have been thrust into a milieu where those who lead them will have many opportunities to demonstrate their skills, or shortcomings. Regardless of future developments of regulation an control, as long as there are hospitals, means to effectively and efficiently manages them must and will be found. For those who will take up the gauntlet, the challenge is momentous.

2 Strategic Management in Health Services Organisations

Like most other service industries, the health care industry is very labour intensive. One reason for the reliance on an extensive work force is that it is not possible to produce a "service" and store it for subsequent consumption. The manufacture of the commodity that is purchased and the consumption of that commodity occur simultaneously. Thus, the interaction between consumers and health care professionals is an integral part of the provision of the health services. Given the dependence on health care professionals for service delivery, the possibility of heterogeneity of service quality must be recognized, both with an employee as skills and competencies change over time and among employees as different individuals or representatives of different professions provide a service.

The intensive use of labour for service delivery and the possibility of variability in professional practice require that the attention of leaders in the industry be directed toward managing the performance of the persons involved in the delivery of health services. The effective management of people requires that health services executives understand the factors that influence the performance of individuals employed in their organizations. These factors include not only the traditional human resources management activities, but also environmental and other organizational factors that impinge on human resources activities.

The strategic management of human resources is ensuring that qualified personnel are available to staff the portfolio of business units that will be operated by the organization. This book explains and illustrates the methods and practices that can be used to increase the probability that competent personnel will be available to provide the services delivered by the organization and that these personnel will perform necessary tasks appropriately. Implementing these methods and practices means that requirements for positions must be determined, qualified persons must be recruited and selected, employees must be trained and developed to meet future organizational needs, and adequate rewards must be provided to attract and retain top performers.

Of course, these functions are performed within the context of the overall activities of the organization. They are influenced or constrained by the environment, the mission and strategies that are being pursued, the structure of the organization, and the behavioural systems indigenous to the institution. To manage human resources strategically, health care executives must understand the relationships that exist among these important organizational components and the human resources functions so that appropriate methods can be selected to accomplish the objectives in service delivery desired by the organization.

The next section presents an overview of fundamental changes occurring in the health services environment that affect the numbers, types, and roles of health practitioners. This material is followed by a model of the relationships that exist among strategy, selected organizational design features, and human resources management activities.

Effect of environment on health practitioners

Few industries have the diversity of personnel and the wide variation in educational preparation, technical skills, professional responsibilities, and professional values seen in health services. Preparation ranges from 6 to 8 weeks on-the-job training for nursing assistants to more than 10 years of postbaccalaureate education for some medical specialities. Health practitioners share a common duty to provide services to consumers, but diversity exists in the responsibilities of these groups.

The numbers of practitioners and their roles have evolved over time and are expected to undergo radical change because of three factors that have transformed the health services industry. These factors are scientific and technological change, patterns of utilization, and funding for health services.

Advances in scientific understanding and technology in health services have triggered significant change in the industry and in the responsibilities of practitioners. Individuals have become more specialized, since one person or profession cannot possess all the knowledge in a specific area of medicine. This has caused not only specialization of medical practice but also the creation of new types of health practitioners with up-to-date and unique skills to staff new technologies.

The evolution of medical knowledge, concentration of technological capability in the hospital, and improved reimbursement have led to increases in the absolute number of employees in nonfederal short-term general hospitals from 662,000 in 1950 to 3,110,000 in 1982 and in the relative number of hospital employees per patient day from 1.78 in 1950 to 4.08 in 1982. Recent changes in utilization of services have occurred because of a number of factors described elsewhere. Hospital admissions and patient days per 1000 population appear to have peaked in the 1970s after years of increase. The absolute number of hospital admissions and the average daily census for nonfederal short-term general hospitals have declined-every year from 1981 to 1985.

The number of physician visits for all sources and places has fluctuated from 4.6 per person in 1964 to 4.9 in 1976, returning to 4.6 in 1981. From 1982 to 1983 the net income of surgeons increased 10 per cent while net income of general/

family practitioners declined. The expected physician increase to nearly 700,000 by the year 2000 is expected to foster increased competition in medical practice.

Increasing emphasis has been placed on cost reductions and control of expenditures by major purchasers of health services. Since October 1, 1983, 5200 hospitals have been operating under the prospective payment system for Medicare-eligible patients. This system, numerous other organized arrangements that encourage efficient use of health services, increased competition, and industry maturity have led to changes in job opportunities and entry of different types of individuals into training for the health professions. Employment in nonfederal short-term general hospitals dropped 3.1 per cent from 1982 to 1985. Within most health disciplines, enrollment in educational programs has either levelled off or declined in recent years.

Certainly, more extensive discussions are available on the health services industry; the health professions labour force. This brief review suggests that the labour force expanded and become specialized over the past 40 years in response to increased utilization of services. Recent emphasis on cost control and efficient operations appears to be having a negative effect on demand for services, employment opportunities, and number of persons seeking career preparation in the health professions.

Environmental shifts that influence demand for services and trends in the health labour force must be considered during human resources planning. It cannot be assumed that skilled personnel will be briefly available in the labor market when services are started or expanded; thus, adequate time for recruitment and training must be allowed. When services are downsized or terminated, use of tactics such as attrition or employee retraining may reduce the probability that layoffs and terminations will be required. Attention to external trends and proper planning provides for the maintenance of the organizational staff at near optimum levels of size, skills, and experience. It also reduces problems from personnel shortages or surpluses such as reductions in quality, inefficiencies, inability to deliver services, and practitioner dissatisfaction.

Strategic management of human resources

An organization that is managed strategically ensures that the functional and operational administrative systems are linked to the strategic and tactical decision-making activities of the firm. The planning, control, and management systems must be joined for the organization to be able to ensure that the plans developed by senior management are executed as intended.

As illustrated in figure organizations are complex entities that require constant interaction with the environment. If they are to remain viable, health services organizations must adapt their strategies to external changes. The internal components of the organization are then affected by these changes in that shifts in the organization's strategy potentially necessitate modifications in the internal structural systems, behavioural systems, and human resources process systems. There must be harmony, in turn, among these systems. The characteristics, performance levels, and the amount of coherence in operating practices among these systems influence the outcomes achieved in terms of organizational-level and employee-level measures of performance.

The strategic management of human resources involves attention to the effect of environmental and internal components on the human resources process system. Because of the critical role of health professionals in delivering services in this labour-intensive industry, a major concern of health services managers should be the development of personnel policies and practices that are closely related to, influenced by, and supportive of the strategic thrust of their organizations. In addition, managers must ensure that the human resources functions are linked to the other internal design features of the organization. The sections that follow discuss these relationships in more detail.

Organizations and strategy

Organizations, either explicitly or implicitly, pursue a strategy in their operations. Deciding on a strategy means to determine the products or services that will be produced and the markets to which the chosen services will be offered. Once these selections have been made, the methods to be used to compete in the chosen market must be identified. The methods adopted are based on internal resources available, or potentially available, for use by managers.

As illustrated in figure strategies should be based on consideration of environmental conditions and organizational capabilities. To be in position to take advantage of opportunities that are anticipated to occur, as well as to parry potential threats from changed conditions or competitor initiatives, managers must have detailed knowledge of the current and future operating environment. Cognizance of internal strengths and weaknesses allows management to develop plans based on an accurate assessment of the firm's ability to perform in the marketplace at the desired level.

Structural systems

The structure of an organization has a profound effect on the activities of employees. Structural concerns include deciding how task responsibilities will be allocated among employees and determining how coordination among the tasks will be achieved, and these involve two features. One is the formal allocation of work roles to individuals. The second is use of administrative mechanisms to control and integrate work activity.

Implementation of strategies occurs through specific programs or services by the assignment of work to individuals, the control of worker activities so that standards of performance are achieved, and the coordination of tasks among workers for efficient operation. Thus, organizational structure should be determined by the strategy being pursued by the organization, since different strategies require work routines, control methods, and coordination patterns of distinctive types.

The several components of an organization's structure have a strong influence on human resources systems. One of these closely associated with task responsibilities of personnel is the technology applied by the institution. Another element of the structure used to control and coordinate work within or across units is the information systems that are required to assemble and organize data on human resources. A third component consists of the more traditional structural attributes of an institution such as formalization of roles and behaviour, centralization of decision making, and complexity of the institution.

Technology within health services organizations

In general, technology is conceived to include not only the equipment, supplies, and other physical materials required to provide a given service, but also the knowledge that must be used in the provision of the service or in the operation of the equipment.

Organizational strategy has significant implications for the technology that will be available to a health services organization. The decision to provide selected medical services or products and to exclude others prescribes the medical technology that an institution must use.

In addition, the strategic alternatives available to management in the short run are governed by the organization's current technology, including the knowledge level of its personnel.

Once a strategy, and therefore a technological thrust, has been chosen by an organization, it has an immediate effect on personnel practices of the institution. Since technology also includes the knowledge base that is required to deliver a service, an entire array of activities such as job design, human resources training and development activities, performance appraisal and compensation systems, and related activities must be orchestrated to ensure that service delivery occurs as planned.

Structure for human resources management

As previously stated, the methods used to allocate tasks within an organization and to achieve coordination among the tasks are structural concerns. Different strategies lead to different structures. Numerous authors have noted the changes that occur in structural features of organizations as firms attempt to serve different markets or to use new methods and practices in the strategies that they implement to gain a competitive edge.

The internal design or structure of an organization has a profound influence on the human resources systems. In turn, job design is an aspect of personnel practices that is influenced directly by structural decisions. Levels of formalization, internal complexity, and the amount of central authority used by organizations determine the appropriate design of work in the organization. Other personnel functions such as recruitment strategies, approaches to management development, and related activities also are affected by internal organizational design.

Information systems

Appropriately designed management information systems provide data required to support strategic planning and management decision making. Information concerning human resources that can be used for planning as well as operational purposes is a crucial element of such a system. External planning depends on accurate data on future numbers of professionals that will be available for the jobs required by the organization internal planning requires significant detail on such matters as current productivity, employee skills, work demands, and related areas. Information systems also should be designed to ensure that managers have access to the data required to support the strategies the organization is pursuing.

Human resources information systems support personnel activities by providing managers with statistics on the future need for personnel as well as information on current levels of performance and skills or employees. This information can be used to identify types of personnel to be recruited in the future and to design compensation systems and related activities.

Behavioral systems

The actual delivery of health services, the provision of most support functions, the development of plans, and the coordination and control of work occur through the behaviour of people and the processes by which they interact. Thus, the ability to achieve an organizational strategy depends on the nexus between organizational behavioural systems and the mission and objectives of the institution.

The actions and behaviours of individuals within the organization constitute a major focus of behavioural systems. If management is sensitive to the personal and professional requisites of these individuals, their needs and expectations from participation in the organization may be translated into commitment to the organization and motivation to accomplish tasks desired by the institution.

Additional emphasis of behavioural systems is on group attributes and the quality of leadership available for guiding the institution through major change. Another significant element of behavioural systems is the corporate culture, that is, the characteristic day-to-day internal environment that is experienced and shared by those working within the organization. The approaches to leadership and organizational change are a third component of organizational behavioural systems that must be handled properly and linked to the mission of the firm if human resources are to be directed strategically by management.

Professional commitment and motivation

The essential building block of the health services industry is the quality and nature of that patient-professional interaction. Despite the existence of a number of standardized practices and protocols for delivery of some services, much professional behaviour is governed by unwritten norms and reliance on individual judgment. Nurses and other professional groups perform tasks based on training received outside the hospital. Moreover, many professionals, such as medical staff physicians, are not employees of the institution but are autonomous individuals who are not regulated by the normal control structures that apply to other classifications of workers.

Thus, the ability of health services managers to obtain the psychological involvement of professional employees and the medical staff with the mission, goals, and objectives of the organization will be an important determinant of the success that the organization will enjoy.

Additionally, a person's performance is viewed as a function of ability times motivation. The behavioural outcomes desired by managers will be influenced by the desire of the employees and medical staff to perform the tasks required by the rganization. Understanding the influence of commitment and motivation on individual behaviour will assist a manager in discerning the range of actions that are available.

Corporate culture

The system of informal customs and rules that

transmit the behaviours expected of employees in most situations constitutes organizational culture. The quality of the relationship between the culture of an organization and its strategy has significant implications for the potential performance of that organization. Strong cultures do an excellent job of transmitting the values and beliefs of the organization to the individual. Thus, individuals are able to determine "what they are to do" in the vast number of situations for which no formal rules or guidelines exist.

Corporate culture should complement the human resources management process systems. The shared values and expectations that are reinforced by culture should blend with the systems that have been established for selecting organizational members, developing their skills, and rewarding desirable behaviour. It is important that management assess cultural norms and plan interventions as required.

Organizational change, transformational leadership, and leadership development

The importance of effective leadership in determining the overall mission and direction of an organization and guiding the institution through major change cannot be overstated. Whereas contingency theory posits that appropriate organizational strategy and design are determined by environmental conditions, senior management must be cognizant of those environmental conditions and determine the response the organization should initiate. In addition, the implementation of organizational transformation and change is the responsibility of senior executives.

To survive, organizations must constantly adapt. This is demonstrated by the radical changes occurring in the health services industry over the past 5 to 10 years. Managers must provide leadership to enable their organizations to make the transformations necessary in a changing environment.

Human resources process systems

The processes used for human resources management may be viewed as a cycle of related activities. Employee recruitment, selection and placement, training and development, performance appraisal, compensation, and labour relations may be envisioned as a continuum of tasks and responsibilities that flow logically from one to another. These functions must be performed to ensure that the necessary human resources are available to support the strategic thrust of the organization.

Although each of these areas is important and must be performed competently for the organization to function, the importance of theactivity to sustaining excellence varies depending on the strategies chosen. Some strategic initiatives emphasize selection and placement activities, while others require health services managers to concentrate on refining the appraisal system. The association between other organizational activities and human resources functions as well as the contribution of these functions to organizational performance are discussed in the sections the follow.

Recruitment

Health services organizations must have a constant influx of candidates for potential implement. New employee positions are required as market areas are expanded or services are initiated. Recruitment occurs even in the face of limited growth or decline in service capacity, because individuals with specialized skills or training who leave the organization must be replaced and because services or technologies that have been revised or modified must be staffed.

The recruitment of personnel plays an important role in helping the organization to adapt and remain competitive. Employees who have recently finished professional training are the source of information on new methods and techniques in service delivery that allow the organization to remain competitive in its traditional services. In addition, it may be necessary to recruit outside the institution if personnel with the managerial or professional skills needed to implement new strategic thrusts are not available internally.

Selection of competent personnel for new or unique positions created by initiation of services may be problematic. For example, an institution initiating an innovative, nontraditional service may have difficulty identifying the activities that must be performed by individuals to be employed.

In addition, it may have little experience in evaluating candidates for new positions.

A number of steps are critical in the selection and placement process. Job analysis must be conducted to determine the tasks to be performed and the qualifications required to perform them. Then, criteria for predicting employee effectiveness are required, with adequate attention given to validity and reliability of the selection instrument.

Training and development

Investment in the existing human capital of a health services organization through a well-managed training and development activity offers potential for significantly enhancing the ability of current employees will contribute to sustained levels of performance because the technological change occurring in the health services industry requires the constant updating of the knowledge base of health professionals.s The increased competency of the health services organization staff will provide significant benefits to the enterprise no matter what strategy is being pursued.

The changing environment of the health services industry itself ensures that the training and development of current staff members will contribute to organizational performance. Institutions are required to develop innovative response to the competitive reformations taking place today. The providers of health services within organizations need to be informed of the factors causing these changes, as well as the role they can potentially play in helping management cope with change. Information on competitive shifts and marketing alternative conveyed to current employees and medical staff will help these professionals to understand the rationale for fundamental changes that are occurring. An improved understanding should make it easier to obtain their support and advice on implementation issues.

A third factor relating the strategic thrust of the enterprise to staff training and development is that initiation of unique strategies and tactics may call for programs to be implemented by current employees who do not possess the necessary skills. For example, strategies to become a low-cost provider may dictate the use of internal management control methods that are foreign to supervisory staff. Management must ensure that plans for strategic initiatives include an inventory of the skills required or program implementation and must design necessary developmental activities.

Performance appraisal

Performance appraisal is the systematic evaluation of an employee's work behavior on criteria measuring important jobrelated activities. To determine the extent to which work requirements and responsibilities are met, valid, reliable criteria must be developed for a job, and job behaviours must be measured.

Performance appraisal can serve multiple purposes for management. First, it can provide guidance for the selection of individuals for promotion. When advancement criteria have been determined, employees who meet or exceed those criteria can be identified as promotions opportunities arise. Second, it can be used as a method for determining increase in employee compensation. Levels of employee performance can be measured and comparisons can be made to improve the probability of equitable rewards being given for desired performance. Third, performance appraisal can serve as a tool for identifying areas in which personnel need training and development or additional counselling. Areas in which one or a number of employees exhibit consistently inadequate performance can be identified and remedial programs to improve performance developed.

If properly designed an appraisal system complements the strategic planning of an organization because it translates the initiatives desired by the organization into specific behaviours required of individuals. Management must identify the key activities necessary for the achievement of the institutional mission and translate those activities into employee appraisal criteria.

Compensation management

The compensation system of an organization can influence the strategic direction of an organization and organizational effectiveness in a number of ways as identified by Lawler. First, an enterprise's ability to attract and retain conscientious workers is partially determined by the kind and level of rewards provided. Second, a compensation system may foster the achievement of desired outcomes by motivating employees if a firm can link valued rewards to the performance of essential behaviours. Third, compensation systems contribute to the corporate culture that is perceived by organizational members as well as serving to reinforce the structural systems of the organization.

The linking of compensation systems to the mission and strategies of the organization occurs through several vechicles. An assessment of the current compensation systems and their influence on behaviours should be an input to strategy development. Once a strategy has been generated, the firms must focus on the type of human resources needed and the behavior is required to make the plan effective. Then, compensation systems should be designed to reward the behaviours necessary for obtaining desired outcomes. The coupling of compensation to the behaviours required to support diverse strategic thrusts is a major component of strategic human resources management.

A difficulty health services managers face in developing compensation systems is the heterogeneity of personnel employed within an institution. This heterogeneity suggest that unique methods for compensating different types of employees may need to be developed. Variability also must be faced by larger health services delivery systems across facility sites or as the merge of larger systems occurs, across systems in compensation programs. Such diversity means that managers must be sensitive to the need for blending these potentially different approaches for employee remuneration into a logical framework that is supportive of the mission of the organization.

Labour relations

Senior managers seek to retain flexibility in selecting among alternatives when determining organizational strategy. Preservation of administration flexibility is critical for long-term adaptability and survival for health services organizations, especially in today's volatile environment. Thus, development of a positive relationship between management and employees by practicing preventive health in labour-management relations is important for strategic management of human resources. This in because if groups of employees feel that management is not interested in their welfare, they may elect to have a union represent them and bargain for them.

Nonunion status allows management greater flexibility in exercising its prerogatives. Loss of flexibility accompanies union status when provisions of the labour-management contract serve as a barrier to the implementation of programs or options that are being considered by management.

For example, a hospital may have agreed with a union that workers whose jobs are terminated will be shifted to other comparable positions or that present workers will be hired first if new jobs are created within their job classification. If such a facility desires to cease offering obstetric service while initiating new impatient services for psychiatric patients, there may be an impasse. It will be almost impossiblo to shift personnel from obstetrics to psychiatry without significant retraining, and the obvious alternative may be blocked, at least temporarily, by the terms of the union agreement. Thus, the change in services desired by the hospital cannot be implemented without major costs and delays.

Health services organizations that already have unions should consider the future strategic thrusts they wish to follow when they negotiate new collective bargaining agreements. Otherwise, an agreement mny serve as an internal constraint that inhibits the performance of the organization. If the institution decides to follow a low cost strategy in the marketplace, the management team must be tough negotiators, granting few wage demands, holding the line on numbers of workers, and stressing productivity standards in an attempt to restrain costs.

Conversely, the negotiations of an organization wishing to compete on the basis of service quality should reflect that desire. Management should bargain to gain concessions that focus on quality of care such as use of employee assessment criteria that development for job improvement rather than providing larger pay increases. Less stress may be placed on reducing staffing ratios or controlling overtime pay.

These factors suggest the importance of integrating strategic considerations into the handling of labour relations and negotiating collective bargaining agreements.

Outcomes

The outcomes achieved by a health services organization depend on the environment of the organization, the mission and strategies being pursued, the internal structural systems, the behavioural systems, the human resources process systems, and the consistency of operating practices across these internal systems. The appropriate method for organizing and relating these elements are determined by the specific outcomes desired by the managers of the health services organization and the other major stake holders of the entity. Although numerous methods exist for conceptualizing organizational performance and organizational outcomes, the outcomes that might be useful for this discussion can be thought of as organizational outcomes and employee outcomes.

Organizational outcomes

For long-term survival, a health services organization must have a balanced exchange relationship with the environment. An equitable relationship must exist because the exchange is mutually beneficial to the organization and to the elements of the environment with which it interacts. A number of outcome measures can be used to determine how well the organization is performing in the marketplace and how well the organization is producing service that will be valued by consumers.

On subset of organizational outcomes that may be used to measure the effectiveness of the exchange relationship and the performance of the organization involves the economic Viability of the entity. Growth, profitability, return on investment, and relate measures are methods for determining the financial performance of the organization. An organization needs to perform well financially so that funds are available for maintenance of current operations, for investment in new service development, and for return to investors if the organization is investor-owned.

Another subset of outcomes involves the nature and level of service performance achieved. Quality of services is especially critical for the health industry, and it contains several dimensions. Technical quality is the appropriate management of a medical problem through medical and other health science technology. A second component of quality called interpersonal, pertains to the psychological and social interaction between provider and patient. Amenities are a third element, which Donabedian perceives to be subsumed under the interpersonal element. He also asserts that an inseparable relationship exist between technical and international quality.

A third subset of organizational measures involves the efficiency with which services are provided, that is, the level of organizational resources required to produce units service. Staffing ratios per occupied bed day or numbers of laboratory tests performed by discharge diagnosis are common standards used in hospitals. The ratio of the status to units of service provided, such as, the cost for types of physical therapy procedure or the cost per X-ray procedure, is another type of efficiency measure.

Employee outcomes

Therefore other purposes and criteria for the existence of organizations and for determining their level of performance. An organization should provide its work force with security, meaningful work, safe conditions of employment, equitable financial compensation, and a satisfactory quality of work life. Health services organizations will not able to attract and retain the numbers, types, and quality of professionals required to deliver health services if the internal work environments are not suitable. In addition, employees are a valuable constituent group whose concerns are important because of the complexity of the service industry.

A number of measures of the attitudes and psychological conditions of employees are available for use within the health services industry. Employee job satisfaction, commitment to the organization, motivation levels of job stress, and other constructs can be used. These measures provide management with an assessment of the quality of work life in the organization. Besides being important outcomes themselves, these factors appear to be associated with economic performance in that employees tend to remain in the organization and are likely to put forth more effort and to work more effectively if the quality of work life is improved.

Turnover and absenteeism are two measures of employee withdrawal from the organization. Price and Mueller have found that a number of organizational characteristics and practices cause professional employees to withdraw psychologically from hospitals and eventually to separate voluntarily from such institutions. The financial costs of recruiting replacement personnel can be quite high. In addition, the organization loses operating efficiency when new employees must be trained in organizational policies and procedures.

Strategic management and outcomes

As previously mentioned, the mission and objectives of the organization will be reflected in the outcomes that are stressed by management and in the strategies, general tactics, and human resources practices that are chosen. Management makes strategic decisions that, combined with the level of fit achieved among the internal organizational systems, determine the outcomes the institution can achieve. For example, almost all health services organizations need to earn some profit for continued viability. However, some organizations refrain from initiating new ventures that might be highly profitable if the ventures would not fit the overall mission of the organization for providing quality services needed by a defined population group.

Conversely, an organization may start some services that are acknowledged to be break-even propositions at best, because the services are viewed as critical to the mission of the institution and the needs of the target market. The concerns of such an organization would be reflected not only in the choice of services offered but also in the human resources approaches used and the outcome measures viewed as important. This organization would likely place more emphasis on assessment criteria for employee performance and nursing unit operations that stress the provision of quality care and less emphasis on criteria concerned with efficient use of supplies and the maintenance of staffing ratios. This selection of priorities does not mean that efficiency of operations is ignored, but that greater weight is placed on the former criteria. The outcome measures used to judge the institution should reflect those priorities.

Another institution may place greater emphasis on economic return, profitability, and efficiency of operations. While quality of care also is important, the driving force for becoming a low-cost provider causes management to make decisions that reflect that resolve. Maintenance or reduction of staffing levels is stressed. Prohibition of overtime is strictly enforced. Recruitment and selection criteria stress identification and selection of employees who will meet minimum criteria and expectations and, possibly, will accept lower pay levels.

In an organization striving to be efficient, less energy may be spent on "social maintenance" activities designed for employees needs and to keep them from leaving or unionizing. It can be anticipated that the outcomes in this situation will reflect, at least in the short run, higher economic return and lower measures of quality of work life.

Appendix

New developments in hospital management

The external environment of the health care industry has shifted dramatically during the present decade. Among the more important changes have been the active encouragement of competition by the federal government; the shifting balance of power between managers and physicians; increasing cost-consciousness on the part of government, employers, and third-party payers; the implementation of a prospective pricing system for reimbursing hospitals under Medicare; and the growth and increasing dominance of multihospital systems.

The increased competition stems from the efforts by all third-party payers to encourage greater utilization of less expensive alternatives to acute inpatient hospital care. This change in attitude toward competition is manifest by a greater willingness to provide reimbursement for services received in such alternative settings and fewer restrictions on their entry into the marketplace. Among the major alternatives that have grown rapidly during this decade are health maintenance organizations, emergi-centers, surgi-centers, wellness centers, outpatient clinics, employee assistance programs, and preferred provider organizations.

The environmental changes listed above as well as the growing surplus of physicians have reduced the power of physicians vis-a-vis health care managers. The pressures for institutional survival and cost containment have caused managers to attempt to gain firmer control over what doctors do. This has created inevitable manager/ physician conflict in many situations. Among the reasons for the increasing relative power and control of managers have been the need for capital to finance growth, the growth of government regulation, and the ability of managers to integrate technology and human resources.

In addition to the federal government's attempts to contain health costs, major employers have been active in aggressively promoting health care cost containment. These activities have included regulatory approaches to cost containment, as well as promotion of incentive approaches such as cost sharing by employees, wellness programs, employee rewards healthful behaviour, and health maintenance organizations.

Since hospital reimbursement is now based heavily on payment per case there is no longer any incentive to lengthen the patient stay to maximize revenues. The previous reimbursement system emphasized retrospective reimbursement consequently, there was no incentive to provide cost efficient or cost-effective service. Now there are incentives to minimize patient stay as well as the resources devoted to patient care. Prospective payment has impacted all areas of health care management in ways that are just beginning to be understood.

Finally, the growth of multihospital systems has been both a response to environmental changes and major environmental change in and of itself. Such systems represent the ultimate outcome of the "corporatization" of health care. The reasons for the development of systems are similar to reasons for development of large, multiunit national and international corporations in other industries: greater access to capital, easier response to government regulation, economies of scale in the provision of some services, and easier implementation of sophisticated management practices.

Future environment changes

The expert panels convened by Arthur Andersen and the American College of Hospital Administrators have predicted a number of future trends, some based on present trends and some not. Although the amount of money spent nationally on health services will continue to grow, it may grow at a slower rate, and emphasis will shift to ambulatory services, less expensive alternatives to inpatient hospital care, and alternative delivery systems. Both multihospital systems and investor-owned hospitals will continue to grow. Hospitals will have to create new corporate structures and business ventures to compete in the capital market.

In addition, the anticipated oversupply of physicians and the continued trend toward practicing in hospital-based positions and alternative delivery systems will mean for these professionals a continued decline in influence. Indicators of such a decline will include prescribed patient care protocols and increased fiscal restraints on physician expenditures. There will be increased potential for both conflict and collaboration.

In sum, all these environmental changes indicate a need for health care organizations to be more entrepreneurial in order to simultaneously achieve both the higher quality and the lower costs necessary to compete in increasingly competitive markets. The achievement of these partially incompatible objectives requires the utmost care in the recruitment, selection, development, appraisal, and compensation of human resources. This is the subject of the next section.

Human resources implications

General

As a result of all these environmental changes, a number of observers have described what management changes are necessary for success in the new environment. For example, the Delphi study of health care managers by Arthur Andersen and Company and the American College of Hospital Administrators concludes that future success will depend on strategic and financial planning, refined management skills, risk identification and analysis, integrated clinical and financial cost accounting, prudent application of new technology, predictive market analysis, and computerized decision support systems.

In the area of human resources, the same study predicts that the 1990's will be an era requiring considerable managerial ability to harness the talent and skill of human resources in health care. The major challenges will be to recruit and develop competent governing board members, to nurture cooperative arrangements with medical staff, to develop compensation programs to attract and retain competent managerial and ancillary staffs, and to achieve greater employee productivity. In addition, CEOs will need to improve their own skills as they move from managing single-entity organizations to managing more complex enterprises. Among the specific recommendations were trustee training, trustee compensation, incentive compensation, opportunities for continuing education of physicians, and recruitment of managerial talent from other business sectors.

Several other commentators have also examined recent environmental trends and their managerial implications. For example, Pointer predicts an increasing emphasis on cost containment, on doing less more effectively, and on product management, creativity, innovation, and product marketing. He recommends more experimentation, pilot testing, internal venture capital programs, creativity, and an internal incentive system that encourages creativity and innovation. Finally, Robbins and Rakich predict a modified human resources perspective including interventions in organizational processes, creative problem solving, a participative and competitive internal environment, and development of innovative strategies.

Two models for the future

Prior to about 1975 the "Simple Personnel Model" or the "Labor Relations Model" were dominant. Under these models, the human resources function was low-level, reactive, and not influential in health-care organizations. According to the authors, the human resources model describes the present for most hospitals. For a select few—those in transition to the matrix model—it represents the immediate past. However, for most small health organizations such as nursing homes, ambulatory care facilities, and physician's offices, both the human resources model and the matrix model represent the future.

The human resources perspective require an interventionist role for the human resources function, which is responsible for initiating and facilitating organization changes. Despite continuance of human resources acquisition and retention personnel activities from earlier models, there is now an emphasis on synergistic, organization-wide outcomes and a direct linkage to organization goals. Previously, these personnel functions were performed in a mechanical, reactive way.

The organization's philosophy is based on a collaborative and cooperative arrangement between management and employees, in contrast to the conflict and adversarial relationships of earlier models. In addition, the human resources function experiences enhanced influence on organizational policy. The specific activities of the human resources function include employee needs assessment, attitude surveys, job satisfaction surveys, interventions to change structure and task design, performance appraisal systems linked to positive behaviour modification, training in both technical skills and social skills, career counselling, long-range human resources planning, and employee assistance programs.

The key differences between matrix model and the human resources model stem from the need to deal with risk-survival issues. In multiunit systems this means the creation of a corporate-level human resources office with responsibilities to coordinate and direct the overall program as a matrix responsibility to the individual institution. As policies, benefits, and wage systems became more centralized and standardized, their impact will be greater. A new attention to quality will result in an overall upgrading of the entire human resources function. Cost savings should also be achieved through such obvious outcomes as the ability to be more sophisticated and efficient in benefits administration.

The human resources department will also assume a greater role in productivity enhancement. The matrix department will be called on for advice and support in changing work methods, standards, and staffing practices. The organizational philosophy will be both participative and competitive. Employees will have the opportunity to participate in organization and work systems, and they will also have an opportunity to participate in the fruits of such efforts, perhaps through incentive programs. However, they will be at risk in terms of employment security as organizations alter their character to cope with competition.

The matrix model will function in a single-institution setting that is either expanding or contracting as well as in a multi-institutional arrangement in which activities are centralized beyond the single institutional level. In all cases, the human resources role will be interventionist, with the purpose of designing and implementing programs to ensure organizational survival. The predominant strategy should be not only proactive, but also innovative. Influence and acceptance of the human resources function are also expected to be greater under the matrix model.

It should be noted that most health care organizations have a long way to go at the time of this writing to reach the human resources model, much less the matrix. Most are operating on the basis of some combination of the "simple personnel model" or the "labour relations model". Their basis approach is being neglect of human resources or containment of external forces. Performing record-keeping or simple functional tasks is viewed as the human resources role. The philosophy toward employees is either neutral or based on conflict. The predominant strategy is either inactive or reactive. The influence and acceptance of human resources is either minimal or not fully integrated into the strategic processes of the organization. This description is, of course, less descriptive of larger health institutions and those associated with multiunit systems.

Integration of strategic and human resources planning

Strategic planning is described earlier in this book as a management philosophy designed to provide the organization with a long-term collective purpose and direction. The purposes of strategic planning are to assess and respond to the opportunities and threats in the external environment, to provide for appropriate allocations of resources, and to develop methods for evaluating organizational performance. In a recent survey conducted by American Hospital Publishing and Kurt-Salmon Associates, hospital chief executive officers ranked strategic planning as their critical concern, today and in the future. This survey suggests that the planning emphasis has changed from "bricks and mortar" to a new qualitative and financial orientation that encompasses all areas of hospital operations. In addition to the area of strategic planning, 80 per cent of the responding CEOs listed experience in finance and accounting, marketing, and human resources as the top areas of importance for today's and future CEOs.

Zallocco et al. conducted a study to determine the extent to which strategic management and specific planning techniques are employed in hospitals today. From a sampling of midwestern hospitals, these authors reported that 60 per cent use a formal strategic planning process. Additionally, larger hospitals are more likely to have a formalized strategic planning process; 55 per cent employ an individual or a department with planning responsibilities; 38 per cent make budget allocations directed to a strategic planning function; and 66 per cent have planning cycles of three years or less. It could be inferred from these findings that prospective payment has made a definite impact on the type of planning used by today's health care facilities and that the contemporary economic climate has substantially decreased the length of long-term planning from the traditional 5- and 10-year plan.

Although this study suggests an increased use of a strategic planning process, it also reported that implementation of the plan was problematic. The process often ends with goal and objective development, but without strategies or methods of implementation or performance monitoring design. Perhaps this is a result of other findings, which suggest that strategic planning is a top-level administrative function with exclusion of middle- or upper-level management personnel or staff representation. Without participation by those it would benefit most, this planning is not likely to develop into an ongoing process. For example, if the manager responsible for developing human resources is not actively involved, forecasting, recruitment selection, and development of required personnel are not likely to occur effectively.

One method of improving implementation is to integrate strategic planning and human resources management through human resources planning, a process that looks at the organization's current and future human resources needs based on external as well as internal environments. HRP involves a plan or strategy to address the gap between what the current human resources picture is and what is indicated it will be. It requires some level of integration with the organization's strategic planning and should serve as a "design and implementation link" for all other human resources programs and systems.

As one writer has commented

> Strategic planning is generally geared to the gaining of systematic advantage over competitors. If human resource strategy is to be maximally useful to the corporation, it must share the corporation's plan. Too often, the linkage is missing. But without it, the human resource plan cannot be truly strategic.

The benefits of linking human resources planning to strategic planning have been demonstrated in other industries. During the 1981-1982 recession, employers who had the most highly developed human resources planning systems linked to strategic planning were able to minimize their employee layoffs through hiring freezes, attrition, and other types of advanced action. Almost three-quarters of the companies engaging in such planning were certain that it improves profitability. It has also been found to foster organizational survival in the health care industry.

Although there are significant benefits to be derived from an integration of strategic planning and human resources planning, most health care organizations are not yet ready to implement such integration. Obviously, the greater the number of "high" values that can be assigned along each of the dimensions, the more ready the organisation is to integrate strategic and human resources planning.

Assuming the organization is convinced that such an approach would be beneficial and is ready to adopt it, how can integration be accomplished? Miles and Snow suggest that the human resources department needs a comprehensive understanding of the language and practice of strategic planning. Moreover, appropriate human resources representatives must continually participate in the planning process to assess the probable demand for their unit's services and to help line executives trace the human resources implications of their strategic decisions. The department should also pursue appropriate strategies on its own to match the organization's business strategies.

Different organizations will emphasize building, acquiring, and allocating human resources. It should be noted that most successful health care organizations will be of type B and will need to develop human resources management systems consistent with that approach. This means that such organization will "buy" the skills they need and provide "incentive compensation.

Finally, the human resources department should act as a professional consultant to line units. In addition to their expertise in strictly personnel matters, human resources specialists should be knowledgeable about organization structure, management communication and control processes, and organizational change and development.

What generic categories of strategies are available to a health-care organization? According to Porter, there are three competitive strategies that organizations can use to gain competitive advantage: innovation, quality enhancement, and cost reduction. The innovation strategy is used to develop services different from those of competitors. Enhancing service quality is the focus of the quality enhancement strategy. In the cost reduction strategy, organizations typically attempt to gain competition advantage by being the lowest cost producer.

Health-care organizations could simultaneously pursue different strategies, particularly in different subunits. Certain strategies are more or less appropriate at different points in an organization's life cycle. Finally, it is crucial that the human resource strategies be compatible with the business strategy of the organizations.

Human resource strategies should be different with different business strategies because the expected role behaviours of employees are different. For example, an innovation strategy requires that employees exhibit a high degree of creative behaviour, a longer-term focus a relatively high level of cooperative behaviour, a greater degree of risk-taking behavior, and a higher tolerance for ambiguity and unpredictability as compared to quality-enhancement or cost-reduction strategies. A quality-enhancement strategy requires that employees exhibit relatively repetitive and predictable behaviour, a high concern for quality, and a high concern for how services are delivered. Finally, the cost-reduction strategy requires a short-term focus on results, low risk-taking activity, and a high concern with quantity of output.

What are the implications of these different employee role requirements for human resources management? The innovation strategy requires jobs that allow employees to develop skills useful in other positions, performance appraisal that reflect longer-term and group-based achievements, pay rates that tend to be low but allow employees to choose the mix of pay components, and broad career paths to reinforce the broad range of skills required.

The quality enhancement strategy requires high levels of employee participation in decisions, performance appraisal based on short-term results, and extensive and continuous training and development of employees. The cost-reduction strategy requires narrowly designed jobs and narrowly defined career paths that encourage specialization and efficiency, performance appraisals based on short-term results, market wage rates, and little training and development.

All components of a human resource management system need to work together to stimulate and reinforce particular employee behaviours. They need to be implemented or changed simultaneously. Failure to a health-care organization to invoke a particular practice, such as broad career paths, implies invoking another that may reinforce the opposite behaviour of that desired. Under such conditions employees may become frustrated.

Enhancement of employee productivity

The Delphi study of Arthur Andersen and Company and the American College of Hospital Administrators identified a number of CEO skills critical to success in the increasingly competitive health care environment. In addition to strategic planning skills, leaders of vision are needed to maximize institutional productivity.

Several of the guidelines identified by Shortell in his analysis of high-performing health care organizations relate to various methods of enhancing employee productivity. For example, such organizations tend to stretch themselves, to maximize learning, to manage ambiguity and uncertainty, and to exhibit a well-defined culture. Organizations can stretch themselves only if they allow employer participation in jointly setting ambitious goals for individual and/or work group performance. To maximize learning, the organization has to have a very well-developed training and development function. The management of ambiguity and development of a well-defined culture requires implementation through appropriate recruitment, selection, and compensation policies.

Health care executives have become increasingly concerned with productivity as cost containment, prospective payment systems, and increasing competition have become environmental realities. The public has become convinced it is spending too much for health care and receiving too little. The era of "open-ended" finding is past. One method of dealing with this new situation is to generate more output from existing resources, that is, to increase productivity.

The principal difficulty encountered by health care organizations in addressing the question of productivity is that productivity analysis stands as a relatively under-development management tool. Most health care institutions have not established productivity tracking systems or methods for measuring and analyzing productivity improvement. However, several recent publications have provided guidelines and systems for such measurement.

Specific management approaches to raising employee productivity fall into two general categories: technical and human resources. The technical approaches include changes with respect to capital investment, new technology, and subcontracting. Human resources approaches include changes in work organization, work scheduling, work rules, and participation processes.

A recent review article has examined a number of structure and process variables related to productivity. Some are related to human resources and some are not. Among the structural factors related to human resources that seem to be associated with higher employee productivity were the use of contract management in the provision of certain services, little or no unionization of the labor force, structural mechanisms to involve physicians in decision making, use of physician extenders, and a close fit between structure and technology.

3 The Health Care : Can Hospitals Survive?

Does it sound's familiar? Resources are scarce, competition is tough, and government regulations and a balanced budget are increasingly hard to meet of the same time. This is not the automobile or oil industry but the health care industry, and hospital managers are facing the same problems. And maintains the author of this article, they must borrow some proven marketing techniques from business to survive in the new health care market. He first describes the features of the new market and then the possible marketing strategies for dealing with them. He also describes various planning solutions that make the most of a community's hospital facilities and affiliations.

Conventional wisdom about the health care industry say that competition is minimal among health care providers. This is certainly true of price competition for inpatient hospital services. Because health insurance has anesthetized the consumer against rising hospital costs, those costs have increase in a hyper-inflationary way. Hospitals do compete intensely, however, for physicians and patients, and new forms of delivering health care may compete with hospitals for health care business based on both increased convenience to the consumer and lower costs. And the more rapidly hospital costs escalate, the more rapidly these alternative methods of delivering care will grow. Hospitals that do not respond to these changes by broadening their mix of services and by developing more flexible distribution systems to bring in patients are likely to experience difficulties competing in this new environment.

Before examining some of the marketing tools hospital managers are bringing to bear on their competitive problems, it might be helpful to look at some of the changes taking place in the health care field that are making these strategies so important.

Changing health care environment

The hospital is the core institutional provider of health care. Yet, for the reasons that follow, as their costs increase, hospitals will be in an increasingly vulnerable position within the health care market. Much like the urban department store, which faces major competition from alternative outlets, hospitals face threats from emerging alternative forms of health care.

Increasing economic power of physicians

Hospital managers labour under some unique managerial constraints in mobilizing their resources. They have almost no ability to control the use of hospital services directly. And physicians, who determine how and how much the hospital is used, exert enormous power in allocating resources—but the physicians, too, are often beyond manager's control.

Existing health insurance plans, including Medicare, pay many physicians fees regardless of where they hospitalize their patients. Thus in most cases the hospital manager has no control over physician income. Recruitment retention and management of physicians—who, like a "sales force", bring in patients—are the key marketing issues for hospital managers. Physicians also have the financial resources to compete in their own offices with many hospital services. Since the overhead in an office setting is much lower than in a hospital, they can frequently undersell hospitals for the same services and will do so increasingly in the future.

New forms of health care delivery

Because of advances in drug therapy and in technology many patients can now received health care without being hospitalized on a long-term basis. Standards of medical practice are changing as well. Many types of emergency can now be managed outside the hospital. Also, many types of surgery can now be performed on an outpatients basis.

All the new forms of care have in common the substitution of outpatient for inpatient care, with both lowered costs and increased convenience for patients. As such, they threaten to reduce use of the hospital's key inpatient services. The extent of the shift to alternative forms of health care was revalued by a recent Blue Cross study that showed in 18.6% decline in inpatient days of care and a 137.6% increase in outpatient visits among Blue Cross subscribers between 1968 and 1978.

Prepaid health plans

More than 6.3 million Americans are now enrolled in health maintenance organization plans. Patterned after the successful corporate health plan sponsored by Kaiser Industries, HMOs provide all their members, health care for a fixed, predetermined fee. Because HMOs can effectively reduce hospitalization rates for their members below the level of the general U.S. population, they present a competitive problem for hospitals.

Changing Regulatory Environment

As public concern over the high costs of health care mounts, the hospital industry is rapidly emerging as one of the country's most heavily regulated: in 1976, New York hospitals alone spent more than $1 billion coping with government regulation. While much of this regulation has had little or no impact in reducing health care costs, some regulatory policies have enormously complicated the life of the hospital manager.

1. *Certificate of need.* Since 1964, 46 states have enacted certificate of need laws that require health facilities to obtain approval from state health departments before proceeding with building programs. With the enactment of the National Health Planning and Resource Development Act of 1974, the federal government

threw its weight behind these state laws and devoted itself to restricting further growth in hospitals and reducing excess bed capacity.

In late May, the Carter administration accelerated these efforts by proposing that no federal funding, whether direct or indirect, be provided for projects in "overbedded" areas.

These restrictions have created incentives for hospital managers to compete more aggressively with neighbouring facilities. The 1977 National Guidelines for Health Planning set a target occupancy rate of 80% for all nonfederal, acute care hospitals in the United States. Under continued cost pressures, states may deny hospitals permission to renovate, replace, or equip themselves unless they meet occupancy standards. Hospitals that do not meet occupancy standards would then have difficulty keeping up with changes in medical technology, altering their mix of services, and recruiting or retaining medical staffs.

2. *Health manpower policy.* During the 1960s, Congress instituted loan programs for students pursuing health careers and grant programs for medical, dental, and other health profession schools to increase student enrollment. But federal policymakers in the Department of Health and Human services-formerly Health, Education, and Welfare—and the Office of Management and Budget are now convinced that the demand for physician services is virtually limitless and increases proportionately to the supply of

physicians. Accordingly, they believe that there are too many physicians and that they area maldistributed by specially and geographic are. Based largely on this thinking, the Carter administration proposed in its fiscal year 1980 budget to discontinue capitation grants to medical, dental, and other health profession schools.

Also, in the Health Profession Educational Assistance Act of 1976, Congress restricted sharply the further entry into the United States of foreign-trained physicians who come for residency training and who, as a rule, remain to practice here.

Reductions in the total number of new physicians will present managers of hospitals in the rural Midwest, West, and South and some inner-city areas—which have very low rations of physicians to population-with problems in attracting staff if their share of the physician market remains constant. Efforts of these institutions to substitute nurses and other allied health professionals for the lost foreign-trained physicians are likely to founder in an increasingly tight nursing and paraprofessional marketplace.

3. *Federal Trade Commission.* While Congress and HHS want to cap the growth in physician supply, the FTC has conducted an investigation to determine whether the medical profession's control over medical school accreditation constitutes a conspiracy in restraint of trade, apparently believing that more physicians would mean lower health care costs.

Under the theory that increased advertising would encourage price competition among physicians and reduce the costs, the FTC also acted in October 1979 to lift medical society restrictions on physician advertising. This explicitly countered HHS's prohibition against institutional providers—such as hospitals, nursing homes, and home health care agencies under the medicare program—engaging in advertising and other marketing practices that might artificially stimulate use of their services.

4. *Cost containment.* The Carter administration's frontal attack on rising hospital costs was blunted last fall by a decisive defeat in the House of Representatives. If passed, the Carter bill would have regulated hospital revenue increases per admission without simultaneously capping hospital admissions. This regulation could crate heightened competition for patients who would not have entered the health care system otherwise, unintentionally increasing overall health outlays.

In a regulatory environment as confused as the present health policy arena appears to be, the consequences of regulatory strategies often have an effect exactly opposite to that intended.

Regulatory approaches to hospital cost containment have, perhaps unwittingly, focused too much managerial attention on increasing or maintaining levels of hospital use and market share. By making certificate of need and rate review decisions contingent on those levels in overall health outlays may actually increase. Regulatory pressures have intensified to the point where some health care executives argue that takeover of the industry by large health corporations is inevitable. Ultimately, the problem of hospital costs may be solved by substitution rather than by capping or other direct regulatory action.

The message to hospital managers is unambiguous: analyze and adapt to the changing health care markets or face financial difficulties or absorption. Now let us look at some strategies for dealing with the changes.

Strategies response to the new environment

Many of the strategies managers can use to confront to confront the new environment are easily recognizable as those corporations use for protecting an enterprise's position in a maturing market. But these strategies represent a departure from conventional methods of hospital management. They include:

1. Compete aggressively for physicians.
2. Diversify out of acute inpatient care into a broader mix of medical services.
3. Develop captive distribution systems to control patient flow.
4. Promote the institution's services.

In what follows I discuss these strategies as well as some emerging new forms of organizational structure that may also represent creative responses to the new competitive environment.

Compete for physician

Since the key to hospital use is an active, committed medical staff, recruiting and retaining physicians are the most important marketing issues facing hospital managers. Because it frequently involves commitments to program changes or acquisition of facilities or equipment, physician recruitment is expensive. Administrators may have to guarantee compensation regardless of direct productivity- for example, to physician beginning their practices. Some academic health centers, the cost of single recruitment may exceed $ 10 million

Excellent examples of both strategies as part of an institution's master plan can be found at Rush-Presbyterian-St.Luke's Hospital and Medical Center in Chicago. Rush constructed offices that house more than 200 physicians adjacent to the hospital. Thorough Rush owns the building, it leases it to the group practices; the lease costs are part of the physicians fees. The private practices of many of its voluntary staff are carried out in the building, which has its own ancillary laboratory and radiology facilities, as well as facilities for outpatient surgery.

Rush also developed a network of community-based outpatient facilities under separate incorporation from the parent hospital. The Mile Square Health Center, Inc., named for the mile square area of inner city around the hospital, delivers 125,000 visits of care annually. The center is affiliated with the Medical College at Rush, which provides academic appointments and teaching opportunities for the center's salaried medical staff.

Having put these two structure in place, Rush closed its hospital based outpatient department, relying on these two captive but corporately independent distribution systems, its emergency room, and extensive referrals from physicians in the Chicago area to fill its hospital. One drawback to these strategies is that, under, cost reimbursement, closing an outpatient department means inpatient overhead costs cannot be spread over as many cost centers, and they inflate artificially.

Outpatient Surgery. Another major development in outpatient care is the growing acceptance of outpatient, or day, surgery. As many as 20% to 40% of all surgical procedures can be performed this way, saving one to three days of high-cost hospitalization. And many patients prefer day surgery because it minimizes time away from work and is more convenient that a longer hospital stay.

Both hospitals and private physicians have established day surgery programs that provide all the logistical support for surgery. Patients are prepared in their physicians' offices in advance of the visit. They come in the morning for surgery, spend the day recuperating in the facility—frequently with friends or family present—and go home in the evening.

Shifts within the hospital to day surgery programs may radically reduce a hospital's inpatient use. Hospitals with less than peak surgical bed occupancy or without a waiting line for elective surgical procedures should proceed with extreme caution in developing such programs. In some cases, however, the institution may not have a choice. For example, the creation or an outpatient surgical program in a physician's office across the street from the Good Samaritan Hospital of Phoenix forced the hospital to develop a similar program.

It is likely that regulators and insurers will accelerate the rapid development of such programs by refusing to reimburse hospital for inpatient costs for surgical procedures that could be performed on an outpatient basis. Ultimately, hospitals may have no choice but to create their own day surgery programs to preserve their shares of the surgical market.

Freestanding Emergency Rooms. Yet another significant innovation in health care delivery could threaten a key feeder system for many hospitals—the hospital emergency room, which typically provides from 15% to 30% of hospital admissions. Many patients who are not acutely ill but who have no physician or other means of getting care use emergency rooms. In many underserved areas, as may as two-thirds of the visits many be nonemergency cases. Emergency rooms are the health system's current answer to the need for episodic health care.

For reasons of both high cost and potential substitution, hospital emergency rooms are vulnerable to replacement by innovative alternative methods such as the freestanding emergency room. According to study conducted for the Robert Wood Johnson Foundation,. 55 such facilities existed in the United States in late 1978. They can provide most of the services of a hospital-based emergency room except for full-scale surgery that requires general anesthesia. Most of them have their own laboratory and radiology facilities, though some contract with others for these services if rapid turnaround on tests is available nearby. They bill as if they were either emergency rooms or doctors' offices, usually at half or less of the prevailing emergency room visit charge.

In the Chicago area, a fresh enter into this market is the brainchild of a former partner of Arthur Young & Company. Dr. Bruce Flashner. Its name, the Doctor's Emergency Officenter, expresses cogently its hybrid private physician/emergency room nature. It is, however, reimbursed by Blue Shield as a doctor's office.

The Officenter operates on a no-appointment basis and, six months after opening, receives an average of 50 visits a day. Dr. Flashner encountered difficulties with anxious physicians in the Arlington Heights community, where the facility is located, until it became clear that he did not intend to build a practice through the center. Instead, its physicians return patients to their family doctors for continuing care or refer them to specialists for complex conditions. In addition to a single doctor per shift, the center has two paraprofessionals who are trained to handle billing, laboratory and radiology work, and other matters. The Officenter required almost no initial capital outlay: facility and equipment were leased, and the capital cost of the leases was less than $100,000.

Bridging the gap between the expensive, frequently impersonal hospital emergency room and the private physician's office, facilities like this represent a competitive threat to both. Hospitals that are competing for patients will offer preferential admitting privileges for patients coming from them. It may actually be easier to be admitted through a freestanding facility than through the hospital's own emergency room.

In Phoenix, the Samaritan Health Service, one of the nation's most successful voluntary multihospital systems, established a captive freestanding emergency facility in the far eastern suburbs. The facility feeds the easternmost satellite hospital in the Samaritan group with emergency cases requiring hospitalization. It was established in a developing area to provide Samaritan with a medical presence that could form the nucleus of a hospital if population growth were to continue at the current rate. Captive facilities give the hospital control over the geographic origins of patients coming into its facility and a low-cost method of entering new or developing markets.

Health Maintenance Organizations. Freestanding emergency rooms occupy one end of a continuum of medical treatment that runs from acute episodic care to continuing primary car. The HMO-of which there are approximately 165 in the United States—occupies the other end. HMOs provide complete health care to a stable population of enrolled patients for a fixed arrival fee. They are integrated vertically, offering preventive and acute care, outpatient and impatient care.

Paul M. Ellwood, Jr. the executive director of Interstudy of Minneapolis and one of the main figures in the development of HMOs, and Michael E. Herbert described HMOs underlying principles as risk sharing and enrollment of consumers. The risk-sharing feature means that to the HMO, sickness is a cost. Since HMOs assume the cost of treating illness, they and their patients share an economic incentive to minimize it. The enrollment procedure ensures that the organization, not consumers or doctors, will control the resource allocation process required to meet the health care needs of its members.

The HMOs embody a mechanism and incentives to ration expensive services such as inpatient care. This rationing can reduce levels of use of hospital services from 10% to 40% below those of traditional fee-for service treatment.

Health maintenance organisations reduce health costs through programs, including an initial screening and periodic physical examinations, to prevent or avoid illness. Just as the HMO is a competitive threat to conventional office practice, it is a threat to the hospital, since its interests run directly counter to the hospital manager's imperative to maintain his or her level of use.

A few progressive larger hospitals, such as Rush-Presbyterian-St.Luke's Hospital and Medical Center and Michael Reese Hospital and Medical Center in Chicago, have established HMOs based at their institutions. The Reese HMO grew out of demands by hospital labour unions for a more progressive health care system. While the HMO uses Reese for its hospitalization, the relatively expensive 1,000-bed teaching hospital setting has created major economic incentives for the HMO to hospitalize patients for routine illness in less expensive community-based institutions.

If a captive HMO is to successfully meet its economic objectives and minimize its fee levels, powerful incentives to lessen reliance on the parent hospital are created. The inherent conflict of interest for the hospital has caused HHS to discourage captive HMOs through its regulations governing federal subsidies. The development of an HMO is a risky undertaking that places a premium on accurate estimates of the market and on rates of enrollment. Achieving federal accreditation is a major bureaucratic hurdle. But certification opens up access to federal funding and market opportunities.

While the HMO holds tremendous promise for reducing health care costs in an open market, it is a questionable growth strategy for the hospital manager. Ellwood and Herbert's estimate—that an HMO must enroll 100,000 people before it can generate a high enough level of use to support a 200-bed hospital is still reasonable. The size of the necessary enrollment base suggests that HMOs may not be an effective way to increase or sustain levels of hospital use.

Screening Programs. Many hospitals now offer screening programs through schools and employers or to the general community for a variety of illnesses—such as diabetes, cancer, glaucoma, hypertension, and vision and hearing deficiencies—that may introduce new patients to their systems. These programs, staffed by physicians or by a combination of physicians and nurses, can be located in schools, shopping centers, or in the hospitals themselves. The latter approach is useful for exposing the exposing the public to new facilities or programs. Sponsorship of screening programs also gives hospitals access to public service announcement—in effect, free advertising of their services.

Develop distribution systems

Many hospitals have gone further than diversifying their mix of services to ensure a more effective distribution system and have developed transportation services to bring in patients. One of the most elaborate of these serves the University of Iowa Hospitals and Clinics, a 1,100-bed facility in Iowa City, a town of approximately 60,000 people. To survive, the hospital cannot rely on patients from Iowa City alone but must reach out to the entire state and region. The hospitals developed and fleet of Checker limousines that can be dispatched from Iowa City to any location in the state to bring patients to the hospitals.

This service has made it more convenient for Iowa physicians to use the tertiary facilities at the University of Iowa which is the tertiary medical center or the start. In addition, the hospitals own and operate an emergency helicopter service that is linked to the trauma center, which can dispatch a helicopter and put paramedical personnel into remote accident sites with in minutes.

Another institution that has made a considerable investment in transportation systems is the Samaritan Health Service of Pheonix. Samaritan operates of fixed wing air ambulance that brings patients in from the isolated regions of northern Arizona and New Mexico. The plane is equipped with life support equipment and carries a critical care nurse in radio contact with the hospital so he or she can consult about and monitor the patients condition. In addition, Samaritan operates several mobile intensive care vans that transport patients requiring sophisticated diagnostic procedures from the service community based facilities to Good Samartian Hospital in central Phoenix, Patients are then sent back to their own hospital with the test results. This system has increased the use of Good Samaritan CAT scanner as well as other complex diagnostic equipment. Though the mobile vans are operated at a small net subsidy by the hospital, the charges from the increased use of ancillary hospital services more than cover the cost of operation.

Hospitals contemplating development of transportation services may expose themselves to common carrier regulation and require special licenses from city agencies. They may also face some political problems from taxi and ambulance companies, which have considerable leeway in where they take a critically ill patient and may retaliate. For these reasons, Samaritan explicity links its mobile vans to its network on facilities and does not pick up patients at other hospitals or at their homes. Nevertheless, escaping the geographic constraints of a physical plant and holds much promise.

Promotion of services

In August 1997, when the American Hospital Association issued standards for responsible use of advertising by hospitals, the hospital Industry entered a new era. The guidelines state:

The guidelines themselves warn against political advertising comparative references to other institutions, claims for performance or promotion of individual physicians,. While these guidelines discourage some of the more aggressive promotional strategies used in private industry, they do give hospitals considerable latitude in promotioning their services

Many of the larger institutions in the Chicago area have placed in the sunday Chicago tribune expensive full colour supplements that stress the range and depth of their services. The supplements are supposed to either highlight new services and new facilities or enhance the institution community image. To avoid difficulties with the federal government over the reimbursement of these costs under Medicare and Medicaid, hospital administrators financed their promotional efforts through voluntary contribution from affiliated charitable foundations.

Michael Reese Hospital and Medical Center pursued another, better focused promotional strategy, Reese arranged with utility and insurance companies in Chicago to include health education brochures developed by the hospital in their billings and other mailings. The brochure were low-key tasteful and humorous and focused on such specific medical problems as stress, hypertension smoking and lack of physical fitness.

Sometimes including self rating scales to interest readers, as well as suggestions about when it might be advisable to seek medical attention, the brochures usually referred other appropriate clinical department one should visit at the hospital but stopped considerably short of directly soliciting business.

Both these promotional strategies are nonetheless, indirect methods of increasing levels of hospital use. Though they may generate patient inquiries, promotional campaigns will never replace the physician as the principal pathway to the hospitals services. It is exceptionally difficult to measure the impact of broadly based promotions on levels of use and such approaches may not be the most cost effective way of reaching specific markets. However, the less tangible benefit of assisting in health education and community service should not be overlooked in a regulatory climate that is generally hostile to institutional providers.

A more focussed promotional strategy has recently been employed by Northwestern Memorial Hospital in Chicago. It has developed a direct patient inquiry line staffed by a registered nurse who responds to patient complaints about medical problems and directs patients to medical specialist on Northwestern staff. The inquirers are sent literature that promotes the specialty sections of the medical staff and lists the members of the section and their office telephone numbers. Although this direct marketing of tertiary services may bring in more patients to see specialty physicians, it does have the drawback of bypassing the family physician who generally mediates between the patient and specialist in complex medical matters.

To encourage physicians to refer patients to the specialty medical staff a critical problem in teaching hospitals, the University of Chicago is developing an incoming WATS line that area physicians can use to contact the university's specialists. A detailed direction of the medical specialities represented on the medical staff and the disease categories where the staff is particularly strong will be distributed through university organized continuing medical education programs conducted in community hospitals. In all of these efforts, the promotional appeal is targeted to reach the decision makers who govern the flow of patients into the health care system.

A more controversial approach to advertising hospital service attracted national attention in 1977. Because neither patients nor physicians choose to use hospitals during weekends if they can avoid it, many hospitals have wide swings in their levels of use. In television, radio, and local news-paper advertising, Sunrise Hospital of Las Vegas offered as 5.25% cash rebate to patients who entered the hospital on Friday or Saturday. The program produced more than a 30% increase in admission during the period. When insurance companies began deducting the 5.25% from their reimbursement of the hospital however, Sunrise withdrew the rebate promotion and instead advertised a contest—a Mediterranean cruise for two for weekend patient. This approach drew a sharp rebuke from the secretary of HEW as an example of profligate hospital spending.

The growing use of commercial advertising by health care facilities has attracted the attention of the federal government. In the spring of 1979, the Health care Financing Administration of HEW reinforced earlier rulings in a letter to its "fiscal intermediaries," the corporation that process medicare claims and audit providers of medicare services. The clear intention of the regulations is to avoid underwriting an expense "which seeks to increase patient utilization of the providers' facilities," thereby increasing the costs of medicare of medicaid programs. The regulations are so rigorous they even forbid reimbursement for larger types face listing in local telephone directories.

Hospitals are newcomers to the advertising world. Yet as competitive pressures intensity, manager are likely to use advertising ever more heavily a marketing tool. Since most hospitals are small, it is unlikely that individual institutions will be able to support significant advertising expenses, and so they should concentrate on the most effective use of their limited funds. Promotional approaches that introduce new services or promote specific existing services are likely to prove the most fruitful. The national proprietary hospital chains will probably begin to advertise their hospitals nationally to establish product differentiation in the mass market.

Structural innovation

Seven years ago, Ellwood and Herbert characterized the health care industry as a poorly organized collection of 150,000 separate units of production that lacked bot horizontal and vertical integration. Many of the approaches I have suggested advocate strategies of vertical integration through diversification into nonacute health care and of capturing and controlling more of the hospital's patient flow. At the same time, however, a major changes are taking place in the hospital industry itself.

Horizontal integrations occurring at an explosive pace. The number of voluntary, not-for-profit hospitals in the United States had remained stable, while large proprietary hospital chains have acquired more isolated local institutions by direct ownership or through management contracts. Since 1975, the number of hospital managed or owned by chains has increased from 469 to 765. The management and financial controls installed by the chains can, at least in the first few years, significantly reduce the rates of increase in those hospitals' costs, partly because the acquired institutions are generally smaller community-based hospitals and are relatively simple to manage. Because the financial and staffing control in hospitals are often weak, they can be strengthened through systems imposed by the chain.

While the initial period of highly profitable growth of the proprietary chains has demonstrated that management of smaller institutions can be standardized and that tighter controls can reduce costs and improve net revenues, it remain to be seen how effectively the chains can cope with the competitive pressure I have discussed. There is no national market for health services. The chains are acquiring hospitals over a wide area, but they are not usually linked together clinically at the local level.

If they are re to preserve their market shares in local communities, the chains will have to develop marketing expects and performance standard to match their successes in financial management. The chins can minimize pressures (at the present time) by selling quickly unprofitable or troubled institutions, but this may change wen they have saturate the market and must still generate profits from an enlarged base. If competing chains expand to the point of saturating local or regional markets, they may have to diversify to the point of saturating local or regional markets, they may have to diversify through direct ownerships franchises into ambulatory health services to protect their inpatient volume against competition from allied local hospitals.

Many of the emerging forms of health care delivery are eminently adaptable to the standardization of financial and management controls and of facilitate employed in franchises arrangement. The parent company could dictate terms of patient referral or follow-up to ensure that any inpatients coming from the outpatient system flowed to hospitals it owned. Whether the chains will invest the resource needed to take this next step remains to be seen.

At the same time, new forms of health care organization are merging that are deeper vertically and more complex structurally than the national chains; they can, if properly organized, exercise control over a regional health care market. Over a decade ago, under the leadership of DR. James Campbell, a forceful, articulate health care entrepreneur, Rush Presbyterian St. Luke's hospital and Medical Center embarked ion an ambitious organization strategy like that of a multidivisional corporation. Located in an inner-city area on the West Side of Chicago adjacent to the University of Illinois Medical Center and Cook

County Hospital, the core hospital contains approximately 840 beds.

The Campbell strategy stratifies the health care system where primary-and secondary-level health resources are organized around the tertiary-care teaching hospital in a metropolitan area. Dr. Campbell felt that through multi-institutional agreements,. Rush should own, control, or link up with sufficient health resources to meet the needs of 1.5 millions people. The organization strategy contains the following elements:

1. *Backward integration into supply manpower* .in 1969 Dr. Campbell reactivated the long- dormant rush Medical College, formerly linked to the university of Chicago. Using state and federal aid to health education programs as building blocks, he built the medical school into a university for the health sciences with three divisions—medicine, nursing, and allied health. By 1979, the medical school had an enrollment of 497. Students. In addition at the post MDs level, 341 MDs are engaged in medical education. Of this group, approximately 40% are retained within the Rush system when their training ends.

The students in the nursing and the allied health profession programs also form a substantial captive market of potential recruits into the Rush system. The prestige of academic programs, including substantial research activities, has helped rush attract and retain a first—rate clinical faculty and recruit top—quality residents to its specialty training programs. The ability to grant academic appointments made it easier for Rush to affiliate with community—based institutions.

2. *Vertical integration with community hospitals.* Using the medical school as it base, Rush affiliated or associated with a network of 11 community-based hospitals in the Chicago area. The medical staffs of these institution received faculty appointment in the Rush Medical College. The medical staff at these affiliated institution have been encouraged to use the expensive tertiary service a available at Rush an to refer patients requiring subspecialty consultation or care to the central Presbyterian St.Luke's Hospital. As a result, Rush has a medial/surgical occupancy are of 91% and a waiting list for elective surgery.

3. *Diversification into ambulatory and chronic care.* During the late 1960's, under separate incorporation, Rush launched to health care systems, the Mile Square Health Center and the Anchor Health Plan. With a current enrollment of more than 32,000, the Anchor Health Plan uses the facilities of affiliated institutions as will as the central hospital to keep its cost down. Patients from the center may be hospitalized either at community-based facilities or at Rush. It 1976, Rush opened the 176-bed Johnston R. Bowman Geriatric Facility for Chronic Disease on its own campus. Although it was intended to care for older individual who are under going lengthily recuperation from illness, it can also serve as a skilled nursing facility.

The resulting structure has effectively achieved Dr. Campbell's ambitious objective of providing health resources for the large population and a solvent, successful core hospital. As federal funds for medical education begin to level off, the clinical operations of the Rush system will be sufficiently strong to absorb an increasing share of the burden of financing health education. The system is not without problems—relationship with neighboring and affiliated institutions have not always gone smoothly, and some of tis operations have lost money—but the overall system is healthy. The Rush systems represent a model of cooperative multi—institutional relationships that link health resources to ensure the survival of all the various parts. Because it does not own all the elements but rather works with them through cooperative planning, Rush is protected financially from major shifts in the market or from vulnerability of individual elements of the systems.

What Is a hospital?

More than 20 years ago, in "Marketing Myopia," Theodore Levitt argued that the price of static definition of an organization's business may be its extension. This is nowhere more true than in the hospital industry today. After a postwar period of explosive growth in activity, aggregate employment, and economic power, it is confronting major changes that threaten its key impatient services. Hospital cost have risen to the point where they are a national political lissue, and regulatory and planning bodies have proliferated in a an effort, as yet unsuccessful to control them.

The challenge to hospital managers to deliver new forms of health care. By diversifying beyond actuate inpatient care into a broader mix of medical service, managers accomplish two things. First, if the activities take place under the same corporate umbrella, they generate revenue that does not depend directly on impatient use of their facilities. And second, they build pathways than can ultimately bring in addition inpatients and open facilities to new a patients.

Hospitals augment their principal source of a patients—the network of office practices of their medical staffs—through their emergency rooms and through organized, hospital-based outpatient services. The expansion and diversification of outpatient services hold the key to a hospital's future financial solvency. In many cases, peculiarities of the hospital reimbursement system will dicatate corporate separation of some outpatient services from the hospital proper. However, as long a there is central organization and direction, through administration or medical staff loyal to the hospital, the separate corporate entities can serve the same objectives.

The effort to capture some of the new forms of health care delivery is not free of risk. High overhead, problems of estimating patient volume and start-up costs and phasing, potential damage to existing hospital programs, and additional bring of scarce physicians and manager all suggest that, at least initially, diversifying away from acute inpatient care will involve financial commitments an careful planning. It should be obvious, however, that the alternative to hospital control of these new health care forms is the net loss of patient volume, both outpatient and inpatient. The higher impatient hospital costs rise, the risker it is to keep the definition of a hospital's business as acute inpatient care.

Both vertical integration and horizontal combination are taking place in the structure of the health care system. It is possible that in 15 or 20 years, most hospital care in the United States will be controlled, directly or through multi-institutional planning, by a few dozen organizations. The not-for profit, voluntary hospital will be significantly challenged by proprietary institutions that have demonstrated in their initial forays into the market they can generate significant profits at reduced rates of cost escalation. Structural changes will eliminate duplications of services in many areas and result in multi-institutional planning where government regulation may not succeed. The consumer, who will find the hospital and other health care providers increasingly concerned with meeting consumer needs, will ultimately benefit the most.

4 Compensation Management

Compensation management is the structurc and process of managing pay. Although effective compensation management is necessary in all businesses, it is of particular importance for health organization. A changing American society shifting reimbursement and insurance systems, increasing consumerism and rising costs have combined to exert mounting pressures on health care organizations. More than ever before administrators of health organizations face a mandate for cost containment. Moreover compensation often represents a major portions of the total operating budget for a health organization. In such a setting effective compensation management becomes essential if the organization is to survive.

Compensation management incorporates two primary objectives distributive justice and incentives for employees to improve performance and productivity. Equity is feasible only if the management system includes procedures for such considerations as job analysis, evaluation, and job pricing. Incentive systems involve rewards dependent on performance but these systems must also be clearly defined components of the total compensation program. A third objective should be consideration of benefits.

A comprehensive program for compensation management must address each of the foregoing areas. Additionally success for such a program requires attention to internal pressures and concerns as well as to external pressures from the general public, governmental agencies and at times stockholders. If the portion of the total operating budget devoted to compensation increases, the validity of the compensation management plan grows in importance.

Strategic planning and compensation

The various components of compensation management are familiar to human resources and compensation management specialists as well as to most health care administrators. However, the philosophy that compensation management strategy should be an integral part of the organization's strategic planning process is not so familiar.

Traditionally personnel specialists have handled the compensation and benefits functions but usually were not involved in the strategic decision-making process. Over the next few years, human resources personnel will need to be more directly involved in both developing and implementing the strategic plans of the organization. Performance appraisal and compensation management are two of the specific functions that need careful evaluation in terms of their mutual relationships and integration into the strategic management formulas of the organization.

Specifically compensation and benefit systems must be strategically related to the overall mission of the organization as well as to the efficiency and quality objectives. It is also important to note the variety of environmental forces that influence the compensation of workers, including the following

1. Tax laws
2. Changes in mandatory retirement laws
3. Social Security retirement plans versus private pension plans
4. Employee attitudes toward work time flexibility
5. Individualized benefit choices
6. The entry of more women into the work force
7. The presence of more dual-earner, dual-career couples who want child care benefits
8. Changing values and norms regarding career mobility

These environmental factors along with competitive market forces controlling market share and profits are all considerations that necessitate the continuous designing implementing and evaluating of compensation management systems.

It is vitally important that health care executives and human resources manager understand the purpose of compensation management and its role in strategic management of human resources. In addition to such traditional issues as job evaluation, salary surveys, and compensation systems, this chapter addresses the key issues of executive incentive programs, physician compensation, exceptional performance awards, and benefits.

A strategic compensation model

Because so many compensation issues have an effect on productivity goals and the quality of work life strategy-oriented compensation specialists will likely become an integral part of future strategic management teams. It is helpful to define a strategic model approach to the compensation process given the relationships of compensation to internal and external environments as well as to other management systems. Douglas *et al.* developed a three stage model for this process. Various components of this model are developed in this and related chapters.

Compensation of health care personnel

Certain principles of compensation management apply to all organizations; however unique aspects of the health care industry require special consideration in the development and implementation of a strategic compensation management plan. For example consumers expect availability of health care—regardless of the extent of the problem, the time of day or night, or geographic location. In very few segments of the service industry does one find such a high degree of consumer expectation and this places distinct requirements on health care organizations and their personnel. Moreover the types of personnel involved in health care delivery vary from those involved in housekeeping and maintenance to physicians and top-level managers. When one also considers the federal, state, and local regulations within which such organizations operate, it is easy to see that the complex environment of health care organizations requires a detailed yet flexible plan for compensation management. Additionally because of these very factors, the necessity for inclusion of human resources management specialists in the development of the total strategic management plan becomes obvious.

Base components of the compensation management system

In developing a comprehensive compensation plan, various factors must be considered. For each position there should be a systematic process for developing a written job design, analysis, and description. Such specifics are essential in evaluating the job and in establishing equitable job pricing. Moreover the existence of specific job design and analysis is essential to objective and equitable employee performance evaluations and determination of which employees merit consideration for bonuses or special rewards. Job designs and analyses for health care organizations must also incorporate such concerns as comparable worth and physician compensation.

Job design

Job design encompasses the manner in which a given job is defined and how it will be carried out. This involves such decision as whether the job will be handled by an individual or by a team of employees, as well as the determination of where the job fits into the overall organization. If properly implemented, job design requires a conscious effort for the organizing of tasks, duties and responsibilities into a unit of work to achieve a certain objective. From the detailed information incorporated into the job design, a specific job description can be produced and this will form the basis for recruiting and hiring an employee to fill that position as well as the foundation for future employee evaluations and compensation schedules. In terms of strategic planning, each separate job design must be formulated to meet the overall objectives of the organization. Where appropriate, each job design must also acknowledge any unique skills possessed by members of a given profession and must incorporate appropriate professional guidelines or limitations for tasks to be performed.

In stressing the need for compensation management to be incorporated into the total strategic management plan, it should be noted that job design is one of the single most important considerations. If each job within a given organization is well defined and well designed, the necessary basis exists for job analysis job, description, and job evaluation as well as for equitable compensation, performance evaluation and employee satisfaction. If specific requirements for each job are not clearly defined initially, there can be virtually no basis for assessing the value of a given position or the expertise of the employee who holds it.

Considerations to be included here extend far beyond the organization itself. Obviously, job designs in popular use in comparable businesses should be reviewed, and general satisfaction of both organizations and employees with these definitions should be determined. For a growing number of health care organizations, job design must involve union guidelines—whether contracted or informally outlined. In addition, each job design must allow for the concept of employee status. Employees with high skill levels can be expected to object if assigned the same job titles as employees with little or no skill.

It would not overstate the case to say that the long-term success of a given organization requires that each of these factors be considered. An excellent example of the importance of sometimes subtle distinctions can be seen in the design of nursing positions. Within the health care industry, the most prominent group of employees is nursing personnel and specializations within nursing have changed dramatically during the past few decades resulting in an increased need for precise job design and description. As suggested above, the graduate of a baccalaureate nursing program is likely to object to being given the same title and duties as a graduate of a certificate or associate degree program. A nurse with specially training in emergency and trauma care has acquired skills that should be differentiated for the skills required of the nurse in a long-term care facility or an ambulatory diagnostic center. To disregard these differences in development of job designs is to set the stage for employee dissatisfaction regardless of differentials in compensation .

Precision in job design is indispensable to the organization for even more obviously self-serving reasons. If an organization is to hire and retain only those employees who are essential to the organizations success there must be a clear understanding of what employees compensation constitutes an enormous investment by a service industry. To assure that compensation dollars are being spent wisely, top managers must have an accurate view of the role of each employee. It is during the job design stage of strategic planning that duplication of responsibilities must be eliminated to be sure that all necessary duties will be performed and to determine the actual skill level that will be required in each position. Care in this endeavour will make and important contribution to future employee job satisfaction and performance as well as to the financial well-being of the organization.

Job analysis

Closely linked to job design, job analysis involves the compiling of information about various jobs, their components and the desired qualifications of persons performing those jobs, It is part of the process to develop concise job descriptions and specifications and to provide a sound basis for job evaluation. Douglas et al. note that job analysis is essential to the development and recruitment of highly productive and quality-oriented personnel. The necessity for thorough and expert job analysis in meeting the goals of the strategic management plan for any organization is apparent. It is also an intricate part of the development of equitable compensation in that it involves analysis of jobs within the given organization, as well as comparable jobs at other organizations within the field.

To return to the example of nursing personnel analysis of nursing jobs within the health care industry indicates that different organization specify varying duties of nurses with accompanying pay differentials. Although "nurse" seems to be a definite choice for many people thinking about future career plans job analysis could show it to be an inadequate and inappropriate job title for some organizations. During this phase of strategic planning, assessment of external organizations takes on renewed importance. Planners must review job descriptions and compensation scales at comparable organizations across the country, as well as those for similar positions in organization within the community, even if the local organizations differ in product or service.

For example maintenance personnel in a tertiary care are likely to confront equipment and standards that are more complex and demanding than those found in primary or general health care settings. Thus comparing job descriptions for maintenance workers in the tertiary setting to job descriptions for similar workers at a walk-in diagnostic facility or a general hospital would not be as valid as a comparison with similar workers in the computer ship manufacturing industry which also has exacting standards for sanitation and a complex high-tech environment. As with job design the emphasis must be on the realistic needs of the organization and the actual work that will be required of a person in this position.

Job evaluation

Job evaluation involves assigning a relative value to each job within the organization. Whether the jobs are within the health care field or in a manufacturing plant the same requirements apply. As Straus and Sayles have pointed out job evaluation is a system for exercising judgment, a system that incorporates the value of each job in relation to other jobs. The value assigned to a given job must be equitable in terms of other jobs within the same organization but it must also be in keeping with comparable jobs in the local job market. For health care organizations with facilities scattered across several states, or even the entire country an equitable evaluation for the entire system will throw some job values out of line with local standards if overall pay scales and the cost of living in certain communities are below the national or dominant levels. In such instances, managers must analyze and evaluate specific jobs even more minutely to avoid both internal and external problems.

Objective and consistent assignment of value is essential. One of the most common approaches to job evaluation is the development of a point system. This allows compensation managers to assign relative worth to numerous positions without discussing specific pay or benefit costs. It also allows managers to distinguish when necessary, among position that may appear to be equal. For example, maintenance positions that require personnel to work in excessively noisy conditions in extremely hot or cold environments or at unusual times may legitimately be allocated additional points to compensate for the hardships. Support personnel positions that require job holders to maintain budget figures or personnel records would be assigned more points than comparable positions without such requirements.

Importantly a point system, when properly developed and managed, eliminates bias from the determination of job evaluation. Job evaluation is of greater significance for new organizations or businesses but to some extent, the changing nature of the entire health care industry calls for renewed attention to existing job designs and descriptions. Current employees may hold with tradition ideas of the relative values of given jobs. But the evolving role of professionals within the health care field—and the most recently educated professionals rushing to fill the newly created vacancies—will place new demands on strategic planners in health care organizations in coming years.

Straus and Sayles note, for example that sex discrimination has to some extent been traditional insofar as jobs more often held by women have been assigned lower relative values. Thus nurses-who must complete training beyond the high school level— may be paid less than truck drivers. Such a system gained acceptance during a time when nurses were most likely to be women and truck drivers were most likely to be men. In keeping with changing social opinion and federal legislation, few such disparities will be acceptable in years to come. In particular the concept of comparable worth can be expected to be applied in more and more areas of health care. It is reasonable to assume that strategic planners for tomorrow's health care organizations will face even greater burdens to assess comparable worth in the absence of work similarities. Although this will represent quite a challenge, it is an area that offers future planners vast opportunities to develop compensation systems with greater equity than has been feasible in the past.

As will be seen when job pricing is discussed, the value placed on a given position by individual employee does not always conform to the relative value assigned that position by strategic planners who must evaluate all positions within a given organization. For example a clerical employee with minimal skills may view his or her position as infinitely better than that of an expert plumber. Because the traditional blue-collar jobs have often been held to be inferior to white collar jobs such selfassigned status may offset differences in compensation that would believe such a view. In other words the minimally skilled clerical worker may be entirely satisfied with a wage below that of a highly skilled plumber as long as the perceived status of the clerical position is not challenged.

Another important area of job evaluation concerns the extent to which the evaluation is centralized. Should a job be evaluated in terms of an entire, possibly nationwide, company, or should the evaluation focus on a single facility? If a job is to be evaluated nationally, should that position incorporate duties not routinely assigned to it in comparable local companies? As health care organizations expand into regional and national chains, such questions will assume added significance.

Job pricing

Job pricing is the final planning stage in establishing staffing and compensation system for a given organization and it involves exactly what the name implies. Once each job has been designed, analyzed, described and evaluated, it's assigned a specific financial value, a wage scale and a range. Because equality across and within the system is vital, job pricing depends on the careful completion of the preliminary stages.

Interestingly, however, in this one area the appearance of fairness is at least as important as the reality if not more so. For example, employees are most likely to compare their wages with those of persons holding positions they deem comparable, regardless of the organizations formal job evaluation results. Employees who consider themselves to be skilled labour rarely compare their compensation with those they consider to be unskilled; clerical employees are more likely to compare their pay rates with other clerical workers, not with line workers or top managers. To return to the example of the minimally skilled clerical worker the assigned price for the job must be in keeping with that assigned to other, probably more skillful clerical worker. Thus equality within broad categories of workers is often the determining factor in employee satisfaction with pay. The same is true for fringe benefits and other factors in the total compensation package. Workers in any general category will probably compare their paid holidays to those offered similar workers, even if some workers in other categories receive different holidays.

Job pricing comes under particular scrutiny in the provision of pay differentials for unusual requirements. Just as a point system gives added value for environmental factors the job pricing system must acknowledge such differences as night or weekend shifts or assignment to a particularly demanding area. Although such differences are addressed during the evaluation stage care must be taken to implement these distinctions when assigning job prices.

Once relative values have been assigned during the evaluation process, it would seem that the assignment of an actual price to each position would be a relatively simple matter. However, the reality of job pricing is a far more complicated undertaking. First of all the entire compensation investment cannot exceed the organizations income. This simple concept involves complex income projections, realistic assessment of the external environment, and a comprehensive understanding of regulations and professional standards governing the organizations operation. Before a total compensation plan can be developed and implemented, the organization must account for all factors that will influence its income and its ability to remain in business.

For example, the diagnosis-related groups (DRG) payment system recently implemented by the Medicare program establishes limits for Medicare coverage at based on the primary diagnosis at the time of hospital admission. A hospital that habitually expends greater resources for these patients than can be recouped through the DRG system could face financial disaster regardless of the care with which jobs were originally priced. To take another example, a health care organization serving walk-in clients would be foolhardy to locate in an isolated area, where the likelihood of heavy usage could not be anticipated.

These are but a few indications of the factors to be considered by compensation managers. Another concern is the labour market in the area of operation. A definition of labour market usually incorporates the extent to which qualified workers are available for and interested in employment in a given field of endeavour and a given geographic region. Differences in the number and qualifications of workers usually vary over time and from place to place nevertheless, such an assessment must be made when determining the fair market value of a given service and the jobs involved in providing it. Thus the entire exercise of job pricing must assume that such homework has already been completed as thoroughly and accurately as possible.

In setting up the job pricing system compensation managers must define such concepts as a base salary that is hourly, weekly, or monthly and whether to use salary ranges or a flat rate. The advantages of such a system are the ease of communication of the wage, simplicity of salary planning, ease of cost analysis, and the defensibility of equal treatment by position and job title. The most obvious and problematic aspect of such an approach is that each employee with the same title receives the same base pay regardless of justifications for differences.

A pay range system involves setting minimum and maximum pay levels for each job title. Such a system has several advantages; No qualified incumbent will fall below a specified level of pay better qualified employees can justifiably be paid high wages; a maximum is established beyond which the organization will not go, thus helping to control costs; and the range can accommodate fluctuations in the job market, whether within a specific geographic region or over time due to a changing economy. One major disadvantage of the range system is that it may in practice make some positions more difficult to fill. For example if an organization usually fills positions at the lowest level of a pay range a shortage of qualified personnel may make those positions more difficult to fill. If long range planning has been based on filling those positions at the lower end of the pay range, the organization could be forced to choose between meeting staffing needs or meeting budget constraints.

When coming to the actual pricing of jobs external factors again enter the picture. As with the evaluation process, job rates paid by comparable businesses and by competing businesses in the same area must be reviewed and considered. If one organization consistently sets job prices below comparable rates in the same area that company will face on going employee dissatisfaction and personnel turnover. On the other hand a company whose overall wage scale is far above the local market rate may be constantly challenged to meet its payroll commitment. As Straus and Sayles point out the burden is on the job evaluation system to include sufficient flexibility to accommodate internal variances and external standards.

Base pay

The steps leading to job pricing are designed to establish equitable pay scales within a given organization. But base pay is just the beginning of employee compensation. In this chapter reward systems beyond the base pay are often of greater importance to employees. However the base pay is the employee's initial primary concern. As is the case with job pricing, the perception of the relative ranking of one's base pay may be more important to an individual employee than the pay itself.

For example, a dietician who feels that his or her pay is in keeping with professional standards probably will not be concerned with the base pay of a truck driver or an administrative assistant. On the other hand the same dietician may be content to work for a base pay below the national average in the field if he or she is aware of regional or organizational differences in pay across the board. It goes without saying that an employee with several years of applicable experience will expect a base pay higher than that given beginning employees with the same job title.

The complex relationships that led to job pricing and the establishment of base pay for a specific employee do not go away once the job has been priced and an employee hired to fill the position. Thus, it is worthwhile to look briefly at the issue of pay over time.

Just as society changes, so do the jobs within any organization. This may be particularly true for certain areas of the health care industry. As increased technology alters the responsibilities of some employees, the very nature of the work day and its requirements may undergo drastic change. As Straus and Sayles (1980) note, employees who feel that their jobs have grown more difficult probably will ask for a new evaluation of their positions. Employers, aware of the changes and the new demands on the employees, are likely to agree. At this point the whole process of design, analysis, evaluation and pricing may begin again. But such a re-evaluation does not happen in isolation. If changes in the job evaluation and the relative value for one job place its value above others a new group of employees is likely to request review beginning the process again in a different area of the organization. It should be apparent that a payment system cannot remain static; at best, it can provide functional guidelines for relative values.

It should also be briefly noted that actual management and implementation of the compensation system are of greater long-term benefit or damage than the system itself. A system with certain inequities may never be challenged if skilled managers apply it in a way that compensates for the problem areas. Conversely, an excellent system poorly applied or mishandled by inexperienced or inept administrators might just as well be flawed itself. As with each aspect of strategic management the talents and judgment of top-level administrators must be oriented toward equitable standards fairly applied.

Incentive compensation programs

We now turn to the issue of compensation over and beyond the base. In recent years numerous approaches have been developed to deal with motivating and rewarding employees who make significant contributions to an organization's success. Such programs are commonly referred to as incentive programs.

Incentive programs exist to serve two primary purposes: to motivate employees and to reward those who exceed certain, defined guidelines. Because of the potential expense involved as well as the potential for increased productivity such programs must be developed within the total strategic management plan. Bonus systems have existed for many years, but these have most traditionally applied to hourly paid employees or to those producing directly measurable piece goods. Recently, however, increasing attention has been paid to incentive programs for executives top level managers, and physicians. Because of the relative newness of these programs, additional care is necessary when incorporating them into the strategic management plan.

Executive incentive programs

Executive incentive programs, which have been among the fastest growing, fastest changing forms of compensation in American business are emerging rapidly in the health care field. More than ever before, health care organizations and their managers are involved in variable compensation plans. Because of the dynamic environment in health care, incentive plans in health care organizations are being developed or are being changed to link them more effectively with the organization's particular business requirements.

Until recently, the health care industry has lagged behind other industries in the area of executive compensation. However these organizations now find that they must follow the lead of other industries and adopt more sophisticated approaches to executive compensation if they are to be successful. Health care institutions across the country are competing for the highest caliber executives. The health care organization cannot afford mediocre executives, particularly in an environment of changing reimbursement systems, declining census rates, and diversification. Increasingly the health care industry Is competing with other industries for the best executives, and—like the industries with which it must compete—health care is using compensation as a powerful recruitment tool. As the emphasis shifts to performance and leverage costs the fixed costs, of base salaries and benefits are giving way to a variety of incentive and bonus programs.

Executive incentive programs, when designed and administered properly, can reward outstanding performance appropriately and can be an effective management tool in achieving targeted results. When discussing incentive programs, it is important to understand the difference between a bonus and an incentive. An incentive is designed to motivate individual workers and to improve the economy and efficiency of organizational operations. A bonus is any compensation in addition to regular wages and salary. Bonuses are often related to the performance of a corporation or organization rather than to individual performance. If the corporation exceeds expectations, bonuses may be awarded to all employees, or to all employees within certain classifications. However, incentives are directly tied to executive performance, and rewards are related directly to preestablished individual performance targets. Incentives are developed to motivate executives to actions that accomplish organizational results.

Executive benefits and perquisites

Generally speaking, health care organizations provide fewer benefits and perquisites for management than do other industries. Perquisites are employee benefits applicable only to executives. "Perks" may supplement employee benefit coverage, or they may provide coverage that does not exist in the standard employee benefit program. The most common perquisites in health care organizations include company cars, country and lunch club memberships, physical exams, and liability insurance.

Annual executive incentive programs

Annual executive incentive programs in health care organizations often consist of measuring financial targets for operating revenue, operating income receivable days and productivity measures. In addition to financial goals emphasis is placed on measures assuring high—quality standards, as well as on personal, strategic, and innovative goals requiring attention.

Meeting well-established targets and standards of performance provides a return that is greater than the incentive pay out. If the executive targets are not met, there is no obligation for the organization to reward the executive with the incentive pay. For example, assume the total operating revenue for a hospital is $65 million. A financial target is established to increase net operating income by 1 per cent ($650,000) and in return the hospitals top six executives could receive 20 per cent of their base salaries as incentives if the target is achieved.

Financial windfalls representing an increase in revenue due to such factors as a technological improvement should be excluded from the incentive agreement.

Personal performance targets should also be established. These targets should not be related to routine ongoing efforts, but should outline a major new effort that is innovative strategic and/ or entrepreneurial. A certain portion of the total incentive opportunity should be linked to overall organizational performance rather than to strict departmental activity This should be weighted based on the executive's ability to contribute to specific organizational goals and effectiveness. This is critical to ensure that health care executives understand the importance of team effort in achieving overall organizational success. The weighting will vary somewhat from one executive to the next, with line managers usually having heavier weightings on financial measures than support staff executives.

Long-term executive incentive programs

Another trend in incentive programs for health care administrators is the inclusion of top management personnel in the annual and long-term incentive plans. This ensures that management does not maximize short—term objectives at the expense of long-term goals. Long-terms incentives for top executives have already become standard practice in other industries as well as in for profit health care companies. However they are just now gaining acceptance among not-for-profit organizations, hence are still limited in number.

The specific purposes of long-term incentive programs are to direct the focus on strategic goals of the health care organization, to build a balance between short and long term goals, to create among executives a sense of belonging and ownership to assist in attracting good executives to provide retention interest for outstanding executives, and to provide long-term tax-efficient capital building opportunities for executives.

There has also been an increase in the use and formality of special incentive programs. Special incentives targeted for selected groups-exceptional performers, physicians, sales persons and nonmanagement employees—have also begun to emerge in both for profit and not-for-profit health care companies.

Benefits from executive incentive programs

Well-developed incentive programs can provide opportunities for added value and other significant benefits to any health care organization. These benefits include the following:

- Documentation of improved quality of care
- Early identification of key targets
- Development of a strong sense of managerial direction
- Development of a better balance between high quality care and financial results
- Establishment of a tracking system of targets on at least a monthly basis so early action can be taken when required
- Promotion of a team spirit and the understanding by executives that each must play a role in achieving group targets
- Focus of managers' attention on organizational as well as functional or professional goals
- Identification of outstanding performers for future executive openings

A properly planned and supported executive incentive program can pay dividends for the executives and the health care organization alike.

Group or team incentives

Today, more and more emphasis is being placed on programs that motivate and reward groups of employees financially for productivity improvement. Organizations accomplish this by sharing a portion of the savings with the employees directly responsible for the improved productivity. The concept is relatively new in the service industries including health care. However, several very successful group incentive programs have recently been developed and are drawing attention and focus from other health care organizations.

With the present environment and challenges requiring maximum productivity it can be expected that group incentive programs will receive much more attention in the health care industry. Such programs are typically very formal, incorporating eligibility and performance measures that are clearly specified in advance. In addition to design issues, the challenge is for management to assess employee attitudes and readiness carefully. This will take on added importance as programs planned and designed to focus activities on improved health care and unit productivity become more prevalent.

For some time, the industrial sector has experimented with variable compensation plans designed to increase productivity. Most of these efforts have tied the reward to the traditional profit sharing or after-the-fact bonus concept. Others have been more ambitious approaching productivity improvement through an integrated economic system that links all human resources to a previously defined business objective. Group incentives constitute a similar approach with incentives available to all employees in a unit or even in the company The overriding premise of such an incentive program is that the business must produce a measured improvement in performance before any such bonus or profit-sharing takes place. Once this economic reality has been recognized and achieved a team incentives provide way to increase the personal income of everyone involved.

These programs typically target improvements in defined areas, such as quality, profits, service or cost reductions. Everybody in the organization is committed to a set of common objectives to increase productivity and ultimately profitability. The return received by the company is then shared with all the employees who made it happen In addition to the shared reward two other traits are common in successful group incentive programs. First management philosophy and practices such create a positive climate for excellence and must encourage high degree of employee commitment and participation. Second, a system and structure must be developed that enable all employees to become more deeply involved in solving problems of productivity, quality, and service. It has been demonstrated that all three factors—management practices shared reward and employee participation—have the potential of significantly improving productivity.

Trends in incentive/bonus compensation

All forms of incentive compensation plans are becoming more and more common in all segments of the health care industry, with slower growth found among organizations with religious affiliates. These plans are more prevalent in for profit health care organizations but they are continuing to increase at a significant pace in not, for, profit, secular health care organizations. The formality of these plans varies considerably from being totally discretionary to incorporating strict, formal criteria for eligibility, performance measures and award size. However, the overall trends are toward increasing formality and toward extending incentive programs to lower echelons with in organizations making such rewards available to greater number and classifications of employees.

Physician compensation

Many physicians operate on a fee-for-service basis contracting with hospitals or other health care organizations for rights to use medical facilities. However some physicians are recruited and paid directly by the health care organizations in a bona fide employer-employee relationship In the past hospitals often developed individual employment contracts with physicians based primarily on what the physician wanted and how critical that physician may have been to the hospital's overall success. This system resulted in significant compensation differences among physicians in the same hospital. Because of the disparity of physician salaries in existing contracts, internal equity may be a major problem, not only among physicians but with other staff position as well. It has been difficult to survey hospital based physician compensation because of the different forms of compensation and the reluctance of hospital administrators to share such data. Hospitals with highly valued physicians are now looking for ways to compensate them in a more orderly and moderate manner inorder to remain competitive. Many hospitals are now attempting to focus physicians attention on overall success through incentive programs. However the difficulty in establishing such programs is in setting up meaning performance and job content criteria.

Although the approach may undergo additional changes it can be expected that in the future greater effort will be made to equalize and formalize physician compensation.

Exceptional performance awards

Many companies have begun to use incentives to motivate individuals who are particularly crucial to the long term success of the organization. Special compensation approaches particularly exceptional performance awards are gradually increasing in the health care industry because of the usefulness of this method of eliciting high commitment and performance for selected employees. Health care organizations are experimenting with these plans to recognize outstanding contributions made by any employee. Incentives may be appropriate for example in projects with major cost savings implications, or in those that in some way increase the organization's ability to compete in today's rapidly diversifying market place. Special incentives are also being used to reward truly entrepreneurial successes. Such plans are designed to acknowledge motivate and retain critical employees who are not adequately covered through existing compensation programs. These plans typically provide a limited number of awards for outstanding achievements and they often include employees who would be contributions may have knowledge of a proprietary nature or may be involved in special projects.

5 Hospital Waste: A Scenario

Though garbage dumps are there all around us, some dumps, however, are more dangerous than others. Hospital dumps are a case in point. The amount of waste produced in a hospital depends more on inhouse patients than on outdoor patients, about one-and-a half kg of waste produced per bed, per day. Of the total waste is produced in hospitals, 47 per cent is bio-medical waste which is hazardous as it is contaminated with disease-causing pathogens. The human and animal wastes along with items saturated or dripping with blood and body fluids, discarded medical equipment, soiled cotton, plasters, dressings, and surgical and autopsy wastes can become a major health hazard as they provide fertile environs for bacteria, virus and other micro organisms to multiply. Pathogens like Escherichia, Salmonella, Viibrio, Hepatitis, Shigella are prevalent and active till these wastes are incinerated and can be carried far through various agents. Surgical and autopsy waste, if left untreated, can be most infectious.

The list of diseases caused due to improper disposal and treatment of hospital wastes is endless but a majority of them are deadly such as AIDS, Viral, Hepatitis, Tuberculosis, Bronchitis, Gastroenteritis and other skin and eye related disorders.

Delhi has 27 major hospitals. Hundreds of nursing homes have mushroomed in various residential colonies. Besides these, CGHS dispensaries, local practitioners, shops and veterinary hospitals also cure ailing people and animals. These aseptic sanatoriums are visited by lakhs of people every day ranging from sick children to accident victims. But none are aware that the syringe which they are injected with could be from the hill of hospital waste lying as such at the back of the hospital; or that the life-saving fluid which is passing into their veins could be from the bottle which has been picked from some heap and has come back in circulation.

Not only this, surgeries are being conducted in parts of houses and flats of private medical practitioners. All the waste generated by them is disposed of in *Dhalaos* or the nearest municipal bin of colonies.

On April 24, 1995 the Ministry of Environment and Forests issued a notification for proper management of hospital wastes. According to the notification every hospital, nursing home, clinic having more than 30 beds or catering to more than a thousand patients per month must install an incinerator in its premises. No bio-medical waste must be stored beyond a period of three days. No person must recycle or reuse any bio-medical waste except glassware. All bio-medical wastes which are non-incinerable must be pretreated, disinfected and disposed in an environmentally sound manner.

Six months' grace period given by the Ministry expired on October 24, 1995 last year. To see if our hospitals have improved a fresh detailed survey was conducted from November 1, 1995 to February 15, 1996.

Only 5 per cent of Delhi's 2,500 nursing homes are registered. 80 per cent of health care is provided by the private sector. 70 per cent of these are mismanaged and appalling. 0.0001 per cent of our private hospitals like Escorts follow all the rules laid down by the Ministry. Different coloured bins have been provided for different types of wastes. Incinerators are always in working condition. Stealing of any sort of saleable bio-medical waste items by hospital staff is absent. But it is a new hospital and I hope it keeps up these standards in time to come. Eight per cent of the so-called good private hospitals though provide better facilities to the patients than 6 per cent of the good government hospitals, but where waste management is concerned, the two barely differ. Most dispensaries throw away their wastes, which include soiled bandages and plasters, behind their boundary walls. Almost all small medical practitioners throw the disposal syringes either in their garbage or outside their shops. Let's now trail hospital wastes.

Thirty per cent hospital waste is leftover food. Most hospitals have given contract to piggery owners who take the food from various hospital kitchens. While this is a good practice, piggery owners, for obvious reasons, do not take food from Hospital. The food is thrown into bins. TB patients are supposed to have separate utensils as the bacterium responsible for this disease can get easily transferred via the food route as well. Such leftovers are eaten by stray animals and thus the dogs of the area appear to have contracted tuberculosis. There are reports that many workers at Bombay's TB hospital and other TB Hospitals of the country are suffering from active symptoms of the disease.

A major component of the waste of bacteriological laboratories is blood, sputum and stool. These highly infectious materials come to the lab for examination. Required samples of blood are extracted and cultured. The rest are emptied into a bucket of sodium hypochlorite solution. This is then led into the drain. Stool and sputum samples are disposed into the drain without any treatment.

In most hospitals bandages and soiled cotton reach the main bin. At this point they are picked up by the local ragpickers.

Waste managers in hospitals also sell the bandages and cotton to 'gudan' markets in Gari at the rate of Rs 2 or 3 per kg. It is then used by quilt makers. Such quilts are sold from Rs 80 to 100 per piece and are used extensively by slum dwellers and low-income households. Bandages also reach Agra and Usmanpur for making *Durries*.

Careful with the cure

According to the notification issued by the Ministry of Environment and Forests on October 25, 1995, all hospitals which generate 100 kgs or more of bio-medical waste per day must have incinerators. Vatavaran's survey found that 20 per cent of our hospitals have *bhatties* (ovens) in place of incinerators. Fifty per cent do not even have that. They either take the waste to a landfill site (Batra Hospital) or they burn it in the open. Ten per cent hospitals cart their bio-medical wastes to another hospital where it is incinerated, for example Kalavati Saran Hospital's wastes go to G.B. Pant Hospital for incineration. Twenty per cent hospitals do have proper incinerators but they are often out of order (Ganga Ram Hospital).

An incinerator is a highly complex scientific system. And, for the best long-term results, technical know-how and segregation of bio-medical waste according to its moisture content are very important. Different models of incinerators are designed to vapourise different categories of waste, with different moisture content.

When a hospital does not segregate the waste and uses the incinerator like a *bhatti*, the incinerator gets spoiled. Hospitals which have *bhatties* in place of incinerators, can put anything into them and to burn wastes. They probably do not get out of order but definitely cause high air pollution. What our hospital personnel have to understand is that there is no incinerator which can work like an incinerator but can be treated like a *bhatti*. There is nothing wrong in indigenous technologies but the latest scientific know-how must be incorporated to make indigenous technology pollution-free. Fuel used in these *bhatties* can never be regular kerosene. It has to be those petrochemicals which can volatise the waste at 700 to 900 degrees Centigrade. A *bhatti* which uses kerosene to burn bio-medical waste is as dangerous as burning the waste out in the open.

Heat and air to aid combustion in incinerators is regulated in such a way as to first volatise/gasify the waste in conditions of inadequate air, and then totally destroy the waste in adequate heat and excess air. Different models of controlled air incinerators are the best incinerators to get rid of all types of hospital wastes.

These are twin-chambered incinerators-where refractory-lined chambers are mounted on top of each other. Volatisation of waste is achieved in the primary chamber with supply of air in controlled quantity through the twin air ducts. The thermax forced draft fan is the source of air supply for combustion. The heat source is the high efficiency, automatic on/off Thermax fuel oil burner.

The volatised/gasified waste passes to the secondary chamber through a specially designed opening to achieve sufficient velocity. The combustion is carefully regulated for minimum turbulence, thus avoiding emission of pollutants, and the use of a dust collector or bag filter is thus eliminated. Educator system at the outlet brings down the temperature of the exit gases from 950 degrees Centigrade to 300 degrees Centigrade before releasing them into the atmosphere. This is a safe limit for emissions, conforming to strict pollution control norms.

Recommendations for hospitals

- Use of glass syringes-to be autoclaved and used.
- Encourage the installation of more smaller incinerators instead of big incinerators in various departments.
- Orientation programmes for the lower hospital staff-to educate them about the dangers accruing from mismanagement of bio-medical waste.
- Tightening the chain of waste collection at hospitals. Right now there are sweepers to mop and clean, ward boys to bring in syringes, catheters etc. and a garbage collector to remove the waste-tending to promote excessive stealing.
- Vigilance cells/officers in hospitals should keep a tap on the number of syringes used and disposed.
- Stop the mushrooming of nursing home in residential areas.

- Severe punishment for the owners of small nursing homes if they dispose of their waste in community bins.
- If hospitals are not able to make these changes, then patients' families should take responsibility for all the reusable waste produced during a patient's stay in the hospital.

The US EPA in 1992 declared medical waste Incinerators the single largest source of dioxin emissions attributing as much as 53 per cent of all dioxin to this source.

Dioxins and furans are produced when compounds containing chlorine and carbon are burnt together at temperatures above 150 degrees Centigrade, and have been labelled one of the most toxic substances ever produced in the laboratory. They are also formed when incinerators are used to burn chlorinated compounds like paper or PVC seen in tubing, blood bags, gloves and other equipment deemed infectious medical waste.

Since dioxin intake does not produce immediate symptoms and its health effects are seen much latter, its highly toxic nature has been underestimated here. In other countries, intensive research in the past decade points to ample evidence of its sinister effects as an endocrine disrupter, hormone mimic and carcinogen. One instance that immediately comes to mind here is the case against the Gateshead Health Authority,

England, in August 1991, when the daughter of a local citizen died of leukemia said to have directly been caused by the hospital incinerator.

Medical waste incineration throws up a host of other problems: Consider the issue of metals, which can never be destroyed. While some, like lead, cadmium, chromium and arsenic become concentrated in the bottom ash and fly ash, mercury from thermometers, batteries etc. evaporates in its volatile form. In addition to this are acid gases that increase respiratory problems, a specially alarming issue in Delhi, where he stack height is often level with the hospital building itself. While it is argued that good pollution control devices can control the problem of fly ash, as well as some of the gases, this is hardly the case in Delhi's hospitals.

But emission control devices do not solve the problem. Ironically, the better the air emission control, the more toxic is the ash, as all these various pollutants concentrate in it. While ash from incinerators must be specially handled, the study found that it was being dumped in municipal bins and in the case of a big private hospital at the Delhi Ridge, even spread out on the uneven surface. Ash is also dumped in landfills, from where these toxic components can leach out more easily than from the original garbage. Incineration as a means of disposing bio-medical waste is being increasingly reserved only for body parts, and the number of incinerators in the US alone have fallen from 5,000 to under

3,000 in the past few years, often with active support from doctors. Instead, there are several other methods being used to deal with infectious waste, as well reducing the use of PVC in hospitals. Some of the commonly used, and commercially available technologies include autoclaving or steam sterilisation, shedding and disinfection, microwaving and even irradiation. And the most frequently asked question about these technologies is their cost effectiveness. The answer, while emphasising that these are much cheaper than an incinerator fitted with adequate emission control devices, also brings up the issue of the cost of public health, and the installation of controversial technology in the public domain.

Clearly, Medical Waste Incinerators change the problem from being one of infectious waste to a chemical one, which is extremely difficult to tackle. Unfortunately, such technology is being favoured by various influential quarters that remain ignorant of its dangers. Infectious Waste Disposal has been an important health issue for quite some time now, and it can scarcely be solved by fire-fighting tactics. Instead, a system approach needs to be applied, at levels, much larger than individual hospitals. This would mean an entire overhauling and control of the waste stream. More importantly, it would mean not rejecting the body of knowledge accumulated in the West that warns quite clearly of the frustrating and tragic experience of incineration.

Hospitals with big names discard gloves after

every operation. While this might be good for patients, it leads to stealing of gloves, washing them and selling them at Red Fort.

Of the thousands of syringes and needles generated by 27 big hospitals of the city, only 30-40 per cent get incinerated or destroyed. The rest get back into circulation for reasons like: absence of an incinerator, non-functional incinerator, disuse of needle destroyer by the hospital staff, theft of syringes by the lower staff of hospitals, theft by those engaged to operate the incinerator or by those who sort wastes before incineration, and the unorganised sector of ragpickers remove syringes from those hospitals where they have easy access.

The rate of syringes varies in different parts of Delhi and it also depends on the condition of the syringes. Almost new-looking syringes without scratches can be sold for as high as Rs 50 per kg. Second grade syringes sell for Rs 18 a kg. These syringes are washed and repacked in Azadpur or in areas around Delhi and Uttar Pradesh from where they are sent to different parts of the country. Drug addicts amongst the poorer sections of society obtain these used syringes from hospital bins. Wholesale *Kabaris* buy the syringes along with discarded bottles of medicines, saline bottles, cotton bandages and plastic wrappers.

Catheters and intravenous tubes are changed at prescribed intervals in hospitals, since they inevitably encourage the colonisation of bacteria in them. But the same catheters are collected and resold by the ragpickers, hospital *safai karamcharis* and contractors who manage the waste. Infections from hospitals thus invariably get infused into society.

It's not only bio-medical wastes but the sanitation conditions in some of the Capital's biggest hospitals that are appalling. In a hospital in North Delhi, a single syringe is used to inject more than one person. In many of the hospitals the lavatories and bathrooms are always water-logged and dirty. Patients' refuse. blood and phlegm is not cleaned immediately. In such a germ-infected atmosphere, both; patients and visitors run the risk of getting infected by many diseases. Half the rooms in the maternity wards had three inches of stagnant water. The wash basin in these wards remind one of scummy basins. Most have not been cleaned for ages. And in the same basin doctors wash their hands, patients spit and the sweeper squeezes the muck from the mopping cloth! Invariably, the operation theatre linen is washed and reused, but disinfection is not prevalent.

When needles, blood soaked bandages, infected body fluids and surgically removed body parts are disposed in the community bins, it is fatal to the health of the locality. Diseases such as Hepatitis B, even AIDS are caused by virus which can survive for long periods outside the human body, if moist conditions and blood proteins are present around them. And both these conditions are prevalent in the garbage bins of localities where small nursing homes exist in residential areas.

Bacterial diseases like Laptospira which affects the functioning of the brain originates at places where hospital waste mixes with household garbage. Forty-three million Indians today are the carriers of the Hepatitis-B Virus (HBV). This chronic liver disease is killing far more people every day than AIDS is killing every year. HBV is passed on to healthy persons through infected blood and body secretions. The recirculation of blood bags and disposable syringes from hospital garbage is definitely a major reason behind the spread of HBV.

According to a ward boy of one the best hospitals, hundreds of thousands of disposable syringes are used daily and at least 50 per cent of them remain in good shape for refuse. Ever since hospitals enforced the rule of using disposable equipment, many unscrupulous people have made an industry of this spurious waste. Disposable culture, though a recent phenomenon in this country, has already started affecting our soil, air, water and health, but the disposable culture of hospitals can be reckoned to be the most dangerous 'infusions' of all.

Hospital waste: A deadly menace to public health

The New Threat from clandestinely repackaged medical waste can hardly be underestimated. Health workers point to numerous serious infections that can spread as a result. Among them; AIDS, tuberculosis, hepatitis and bacterial diseases. Apart from the threat of infection, unhygienic waste disposal undermines the recent drive across the country to make treatment of patients safer by introducing disposable products. Worse, the medical fraternity's attitude to the problem has so far been largely apathetic.

Much of the danger is hidden. Most city hospitals exhibit the old Dr. Jekyll and Mr. Hyde syndrome-a reassuringly clean exterior and a festering, illegal garbage dump tucked away in a corner. New Delhi's All India Institute of Medical Sciences, the country's premier medical institution, is a case in point. If Dr. Lalit Nath, a community-health expert who was the acting director of AIIMS till recently, is to be believed, the problem does not exist; "We do not have a waste disposal dump at AIIMS. Everything is incinerated or removed directly."

The picture on the ground, however, is vastly different. Instead of disposing of waste in the incinerator, ward staff at AIIMS actually throw it in an open garbage dump next to it. And a contractor, who has a shack nearby, hires people to sort out anything saleable such as disposable syringes, intravenous tubes, gloves and even blood bags. These are reportedly "washed" and then sold in bazaars, such as the one behind Delhi's Red Fort, at bargain prices. A disposable syringe that normally costs Rs 12 goes for as little as Rs. 2. The story is much the same elsewhere. Outside the Calcutta Medical College and Hospital, West

Bengal's main government-run hospital, a huge vat overflows with waste generated by the hospital. It lies unattended to for weeks. Most hospitals across the city are as apathetic. And it is only recently that the West Bengal Pollution Control Board, in collaboration with the Calcutta-based All India Institute of Hygiene and public health, has commissioned a survey to determine the seriousness of the problem. Iqbal Malik, an eco-activist who heads Vatavaran, says: "If we do not do something, we will certainly have epidemics visiting us time and time again." One indication of how serious the problem has become is that many doctors across the country are reverting to the good old glass syringe that can be used, autoclaved-a high-temperature, high-pressure treatment to kill germs-and reused. Experts say that even guesstimates of how many people actually contract infections from reused medical disposables are not available. Without regular compilation of medical records and case histories-another area of neglect-the magnitude of the problem is difficult to assess.

The Union Ministry of Environment and Forests shows signs of having finally woken up to the threat. It is in the final stages of formulating a guideline that will make it mandatory for every hospital with 30 beds or more to incinerate its infectious waste. The Bio-Medical Wastes Rules, 1995, will have other provisions incorporated, including those to ensure proper handling, packaging and transport of such waste. A total ban on disposal of medical waste in municipal drains is also contemplated. Dr. Lakshmi Raghupathy, joint advisor in the ministry, says: "Suggestions and recommendations to our draft notification are being considered and we hope the rule will be a reality soon." Dr. A.K. Mukherji, director-general of the Central Government Health Services, adds: "The problem of hospital-waste disposal is important, complex and serious, and needs to be tackled urgently. The new rule may help."

That such a measure is necessary to goad authorities into action is evident from the lackadaisical approach of various states to the problem. In Maharashtra, Dr. Subhash Salunke, director of Maharashtra State Health Services, claims that the Government is in the process of installing incinerators in the 22 government hospitals. But he is silent about the over 2,000 other government and private hospitals across the state. In Delhi, according to Malik: "Only 5 per cent of Delhi's 2,500 nursing homes are registered, so there is no way of getting accurate figures. But judging from our survey, only a small percentage have incinerators." There are fears that hospitals will get around the new rule. Furthermore, the 30-bed limit for the installation of incinerators can easily be circumvented and Indian metros may soon see the mushrooming of 29-bed hospitals.

Yet, where ever hospitals have approached the problem with the seriousness it merits the results have been an inspiration to others. The Escorts

Heart Institute and Research Center in New Delhi for instance, has an elaborate infection-control programme supervised by the top management. Apart from sorting out waste at source and incinerating it later, the hospital runs regular courses on waste-management for nurses. It also carries out surprise checks to ensure that the system is working. Cardiac Surgeon Naresh Trehan, who heads the institute, says: "We believe it is criminal not to pay attention to the problem of waste-management." Trehan believes that watchdog bodies staffed by committed professionals and NGOs should be set up to help ensure that hospitals are observing rules.

Some, like the New Delhi Municipal Corporation's Charakpalika Hospital, have found innovative ways to ensure their waste is disposed of effectively. The hospital entrusted the task to Sulabh International, an NGO, paying it a monthly fee of Rs 1.10 lakh. Says Dr. V.K. Singhal, the hospital's chief medical officer: "This helped us to curb the malpractice that were flourishing. It is far cheaper, too."

However, KEM Hospital ran into problems when it banned the reuse of disposable items such as catheters, guide-wire pacemakers and heart valves. The hospital was reacting to the Supreme Court judgment last november bringing the medical profession under the ambit of the Consumer Protection Act. But poor patients held rallies to protest against the ban because buying fresh items would have resulted in increased cost of treatment for them. However, as Pai points out. "The fact remains that the practice is irregular and may have serious legal consequences."

Paradoxically, some ecologists have protested against the use of incinerators for burning plastic disposables. These are known to spew toxic gases and countries such as the US have move away from incineration to shredding, microwaving and destruction of waste at source. Since India may not be able to afford such expensive disposal techniques, most believe that incinerators are the answer. What is needed is more attention by hospital management to waste disposal and stricter monitoring of disposal systems. The Government also needs to penalise laggards and violators severely. Only then will public confidence be restored in the nation's health services' ability to dispose of waste without infecting those they are supposed to cure.

6 What is Health Administration

Administrative leadership is an essential, but often neglected, ingredient in the search for solutions to the serious problems of equity, quality, and efficiency in the delivery of health and medical services in this country. This paper examines the major roles and responsibilities of health administrators, and suggests that: health administration is unique, both as a specially field of administration and as a function within the health and medical care industry: health administration may be viewed theoretically in a systems context but must also be looked at as an emerging profession that is taking on the attributes as well as the self-limiting features of professionalism; and health administration as an area of practice has the potential for steering the larger health and medical care industry into patterns of responsiveness, responsibility, and reconciliation.

The uniqueness of health administration

Although health administration's commonalties with other kinds of administration are acknowledged and its interrelationships with other kinds of health and medical care activities are assumed, it also has unique characteristics which set it apart and afford special opportunities for both practice and education.

Most of the unique characteristics of health administration derive from the idiosyncrasies of the health and medical care "industry," one of the human service industries which comprise the larger service industry complex in our society.

Delivery of individualised services

A unique feature of the health and medical care industry is the extent to which its services must be individualized usually to a greater extent than those of other human services industries, regardless of whether delivered in large, complex, impersonal settings or in smaller, more intimate ones. Whatever the size and function of the organizational setting, management and organization in the health field must be combined with provision of services personally designed for each client of each organization. Personal health and medical care services simply cannot be mass-produced and sold, as are the products of many modern industries; even community health and medical services delivered on an agency-to-group basis must be tailored to the needs of particular groups and their members.

Professionalism in the health and medical care industry

The health and medical care industry is the most highly professionalized industry in our society. Members of a number of professions, accredited in a variety of ways work within the industry, both as provider of direct services and as directors of institutions, agencies, and programs. However, all other professionals involved in direct patient care activities one way or another, are responsive and responsible to the most prestigious of professionals, the physicians.

The U.S. health and medical care system has been dominated by the medical profession throughout its more than 200 years of development. Only within the last decade or two has there been evidence that this balance of power can, should, or probably will shift. However, this shift will be neither sudden nor rapid, as illustrated by the following report of positions taken by the American Medical Association at its 1973 Annual Convention:

> While noting that conflicting legal decisions have been made on the question of accountability, the AMA deplored the actions of some hospital boards in attempting to set medical policies, and strongly reaffirmed that accountability for patient care in hospitals is the responsibility of attending physicians.
>
> Among its actions, the AMA in effect turned down the American Hospital Association's peer review plan, known as the Quality Assurance Program (QAP), by expressing "grave reservations" because of "its potential for lay control of medical practice"

Since professionals tend to identify more closely

with professional goals than with organization, subsystem, or industry goals, the major problems of the health and medical care industry receive minimal attention from the professional groups or their individual members-wherein lies one of the main sources as challenge and opportunity for the emerging health administration profession.

Complexities of the health and medical care industry

A third major characteristic of the health and medical care system in the United States is its extreme complexity. This complexity is referred to again and again in the health and medical care literature. The system's three major components—its users, its providers of direct services, and the many mechanisms for bringing users and providers together—interact in myriad and complex ways.

Factors contributing to this complexity are several: (1) the pluralistic, "mosaic" nature of the mechanisms involved in bringing the system's users and providers together; (2) the interface of public service objectives with private ownership interests and obligations within the industry; (3) the heavy dependence upon indirect financing from both private and public third party sources; and (4) the complicated intra-and inter-system relationships which must be developed, rationalized, and maintained.

The wide range of delivery facilities

The industry's pluralistic nature is manifested in service delivery settings ranging from huge academic health centers providing comprehensive care to small single-service units. Between these extremes are a wide variety of organizations, such as teaching hospitals, state mental hospitals, extended care facilities, voluntary special disease agencies, comprehensive health planning agencies, group practices, community mental health centers, solo and partnership physician practices, commercial and nonprofit health insurance plans, regional health authorities, and others. All too frequently, the health services provided by this large group of agencies are fragmented and uncoordinated from the user's vantage point. Such pluralism requires a diversity of administrative approaches unequalled in other speciality fields.

Administrative complexity's also increased by ownership patterns in the health and medical services industry with the predominant pattern still based in the private sector. Should health administrators in the private sector be considered quasi-public servants accountable to the communities which they serve? If so, can they subordinate the interests of their private owners in meeting this broader set of goals?

Financial reimbursement arrangements

Financing arrangement also increase administrative complexity with the health and medical care system. Payments for services are derived from a variety of sources: direct payment from patients; capitation payments, from pre-paid insurance plans; reimbursement from commercial insurance companies, Blue Cross/Blue Shield agencies, Medicare and Medicaid, and several other sources. Such a varied mix of financial arrangements not only upsets classical supply and demand market conditions, but also creates administrative layers between provision of, and payment for, services with attendant delays, regulations and other frustrations for the administrators of health service agencies.

All of the above leads to the need for a very high degree of inter and intra-organizational coordination between units of the health and medical care system, and to a complexity of professional and administrative relationships unrivalled by most other industries.

Some may argue that none of these factors are really unique, and will point to similar examples in other fields particularly fields providing other human services. However, in no other field do all of these factors converge as they do in the U.S. health and medical care system. For example, the welfare system is also concerned with the provision of highly personal services, but these services are rendered mostly by tax-funded public agencies, not by privately owned organizations with indirect payment mechanisms as in the health systems.

Administrative and organisational theory

Administrative roles and functions in the health system are best examined in broader framework of administrative and organizational theory. The brief discussion which follows traces the development of several theories of management and their application to problems of health administration.

The classical school of management sought general principles that could be universally applied to any organization. These principles focused on internal operations within an organization and emphasized strict attention to method, measurement, and work standards. This "gospel of efficiency," preached by such advocates as Frederick W. Taylor, Henri Fayol, Luther Gulick, Lyndall Urwick, and others, resulted in many of the "principles" of management still in wide use today-work specialization, separation of line and staff activities, and hierarchical organization, to mention just a few. Attempts to apply some of these principles blindly to health services organizations are frequently unsuccessful because of the highly personal nature of the services involved and the professionalized work force which renders the services.

World War II helped to produce a broader appreciation of the administrative process as a system of policy formulation, decision-making among alternative policies, programming work to carry out such policies, and evaluation of program outcomes. This model stressed purpose more than method. Simon, for example, conceived of administrative organizations as decision making structures, with efficient organizations narrowing the scope of decisions to be made.

The behavioural approach to management

The behavioural approach to management developed at approximately the same time. The human relations "pioneers" viewed organizations as social systems possession complex values, motives, and attitudes, with considerable attention paid to employee motivation and cooperation using "democratic" strategies of management and organization? The effects of the human relations school of management theory can be seen in participative management and management by objectives strategies practiced in many of our health care institutions today.

The three major approaches described above all focus inwardly on organizational structure, both formal and informal. Rigid application of such approaches often results in considerable goal displacement. The more recent development of the neo-classical, or structuralist, school of management theory takes a different approach. Administration is viewed as a system of responsibility or accountability, with emphasis shifting to external organizational relations. Attention focuses on the responsibilities of an institution to its constituencies and the arrangements by which such responsibilities are met. In cases where external forces inhibit the ability of an organization to meet these responsibilities fully, the organization may take on the role of change agent in the community, working toward needed changes in attitudes, values, and social policy. Accountability is used as a primary control mechanism within the organization, and program emphasis—emphasis on ends rather means—is a major weapon in combatting goal displacement.

Principles of accountability and program

emphasis are beginning to have their effect on the delivery of health services, but they still frequently conflict with the goals of private owners and professional providers in the system. Resolution of the conflict between administrative authority, directed toward public accountability, and professional authority, often preoccupied with professional prerogatives, may be the single most important challenge facing the health system today.

Components of the health administration sub-system

No single model could hope to describe the complex set of relationships between health administration and the many other components of the health and medical care system. However, administrative functions within the system can be described using general systems theory.

In simple terms administration in the health delivery system can be viewed as the process of converting a set of inputs into a set of outputs, with success and/or failures at the output stage influencing future input through positive and negative feedback. The system is an open one, in the sense that the input, conversion, and output components are heavily influenced by a variety of environmental factors—socio-economic, political, and technological-which sometimes facilitate and often constrain the process of delivering services.

Inputs to the health administration sub system are several and include: needs and demands for health services determined through planning, analysis, evaluation and advocacy;

resources required to provide services including manpower, capital and operating funds, and necessary technology; behavioural variables which affect utilization of services; community values which influence both service outputs and the mechanisms for providing them; formal regulations which are imposed by external authorities; and "power inputs" which are largely determined by political processes. Finally, given the complexity of the system as mentioned previously, a high degree of administrative invention is an essential input factor.

Three types of output

Outputs are of three types: specific health services rendered to clients and related outcomes of these services: evaluation of health services rendered and related plans for new and/or modified services: and symbolic messages transmitted to the clientele and the community at large through the attitudes, gestures, and statements of those providing care. These determine the "image" of the health services organization in the community. As mentioned above, the effectiveness of services rendered will feed back to the input stage and will influence future needs, demands, and resources.

The conversion process requires organization of resources into a set of formal and informal procedures for the delivery of health and medical care. Administrative and organizational theory, as discussed previously, has particular applicability to the conversion process. However, it must be applied with full realization of the limitations of all such theories when applied to a set of problems which are largely situational in nature. Furthermore, much of this theory has been developed by experimentation in the material goods production industries, and such theory does not take into account the "uniqueness" of health administration.

Environmental factors

Environmental factors which influence the health administration sub-system are several. Economic conditions influence the market value of goods and labour required to provide health care. Community attitudes and values help to determine the level of resources that will be made available for community health services. Political factors affect the level of regulation which is levied on health organizations in the conduct of their business. A variety of third party organizations representing consumers the "people's health movement", employees, professional providers, as well as third party payment agencies all constitute elements of the environment for health administrators.

The model reinforces the concept that health administrators cannot be viewed as internal managers only. They participate directly in the policy-making process by virtue of their positions as leaders of administrative units, with complex relationships to consumers, providers, and the several environmental forces mentioned above.

The team approach

Finally, two points seem to flow from this

discussion of systems theory as applied to health administration. First, administrators are not the only participants in the process of health administration. System complexity mandates team approaches and shared responsibility among administrators, physicians, nurses, other health professionals, politicians, community leaders et al. in the allocation and application of resources to effect successful health outcomes. Second, administrators are by no means in total control of their own activities, let alone all aspects of the larger health and medical care system, and to date their impact on changing that system has been marginal.

Pluralism and complexity of delivery settings

As mentioned above, personal and community health services are planned and delivered in a variety of settings, ranging from large complex organizations, such as university medical centers, to very small organizations with complex purposes and activities, such as a five man comprehensive health planning agency responsible for planning and coordinating all personal and environmental health services for a large metropolitan area. Hence the complexity of the administrative task is related to both organizational size and mission.

In addition to organizational complexity, health administrators are responsible for coordinating the delivery of a broad array of services, some requiring complex technology and others dependent upon careful attention to personal, social, and cultural factors.

Despite the complexities of the task, administration within the health care system has traditionally been viewed as a function of less significance, and in some way subordinate to, the direct provision of services. In fact, however, the delivery of health services to individuals and to groups of individuals is inherently an administrative process dependent upon planning, allocation of scarce resources, evaluation of performance, and other tasks basic to management. This is not to say that administrators can carry out the task alone. Obviously, team efforts are required involving physicians, nurses, and other health professionals as well as administrators, and it is important to note that responsibility for effective administration is shared by all members of this team. The fact, however, that health administrators do not "lay on hands" does not diminish the importance of their broader functions in the system; an analogy would be to consider the functions of administrators and planners in the space industry less than those of astronauts, since the former group has never landed on the moon. In fact, of course, health administrators must take final responsibility for all activities which take place in the organizations which they manage, and this includes quality of care as well as efficiency in the allocation of resources.

Administrative accountability in the health system

As mentioned previously in this paper, health administrators frequently find themselves on the horns of a dilemma with regard to public accountability because of the competing demands placed upon them. A simple taxonomy of administrative accountability in the health field would include six elements: owner accountability, community accountability, consumer accountability, resources accountability, regulatory accountability, and third party accountability.

Administrators are formally responsible to the sponsors or owners of their organizations, e.g., the board of trustees of the community hospital, the board of health for the local health agency, the governor of the state for the state health planning agency. Administrators cannot ignore patterns of formal accountability, even when the issues involved may be in conflict with their own personal value system or what they perceive to be the values of the public being served.

Administrators are also accountable to the communities which their organizations serve. Problems arise when the community does not have a well-identified representative body to speak for it. Consumer accountability accrues to the patients served by the administrator's organization or program. Conflicts sometimes develop between consumer accountability and community accountability, particularly when the client group is a small, stratified segment of the larger community.

In a sense administrators are also accountable to the scarce resources essential to accomplishment of organizational goals. Resource accountability accrues to the professional providers of care who operate as private entrepreneurs in most health delivery settings as well as to other scarce employment categories and to providers of funds for capital and operating purposes.

Administrators are also responsible to the public and private agencies which exercise legal or voluntarily-yielded control over their organizations such as the State Health Department and the Joint Commission on Accreditation of Hospitals. Finally administrators must respond to organizations which serve as intermediaries or third parties in the provision of financial and other resources necessary to the accomplishment of organizational missions. Examples include Blue Cross and other private insurance carriers, employee unions, and county medical societies.

Administrative roles

How, then, do health administrators respond to this complex set of demands which are often in competition with one another? A variety of role responses are possible including one or some combination of the following; (1) Super Clerk-retreating to the position of one who oversees a complex process of paperwork, designed primarily to facilitate the activities of the private entrepreneurs providing medical care within the organization; (2) Efficiency Expert adopting the role of one whose only purpose is to "optimize the allocation of resources" thus leaving the more difficult problems of policy to other; (3) Magician the Houdini of the health system bridging the gap between unlimited demands for health services and scarce resources; (4) Ombudsman spokesman for the clients or consumers of health services; (5) Negotiator-super arbitrator of the conflicts between special interests; (8) Empire Builder "grabbing as big a piece of the action as possible" (7) Philosopher-King—the benevolent despot, with ultimate policy authority.

The list of possible roles is almost endless; educator, fireman, change agent, scapegoat, czar, and so forth. Although most administrators would probably acknowledge playing some of these roles on some occasions none of them would appear to be an accurate per sufficient description of administrative processes. Administrators must aspire to a broader role which emphasizes proper balance between accountability to all the special interests mentioned tempered with an overriding sense of moral accountability. They must constantly strive to develop and maintain proper perspective between means and ends between organizational imperatives and a broader community perspective. To do this they have to become power brokers; not neutral brokers but "tilters" facilitators of the public interest within their organizations and community. Assumption of such a role requires a high degree of administrative invention, flexibility and change orientation.

Emerging professionalism in health administration

Health administration can be viewed as an emerging profession. Historically the early development of this field placed the emphasis on business management functions with program and quality control in the hands of physicians. During the last 15 to 20 years the era of the "lay" administrator has arrived with current emphasis being placed on the management of large and complex medical care organizations using management and systems techniques. If this fledgling profession is to continue to mature, then future emphasis will need to be placed on extra-organizational responsibilities for assessment of community health needs and demands and active participation in the policy-making process to insure that adequate community health services are provided. Hence, two important ingredients in the further professionalisation of health administrators will be policy orientation and health rather than medical care, orientation;

The history of professional development in other fields is not all favorable. In too many cases, professional goals and codes of ethics which originally were intended to be client-serving degenerate over time and tend to become self-serving to members of the profession. If this is to be avoided in the emerging profession of health administration, members of the profession must continually be guided by Strauss' "3R's"—responsiveness to the needs and demands of users of the health system; responsibility for the functions of planning, organizing, controlling, and coordinating services; and reconciliation of the vast array of knowledge, attitudes, and skills that interact in the functioning of the system.

There are many ingredients for the successful development of a new profession with the positive characteristics which have been suggested. These include formal education, directed experience, commitment, and ability—all parts of professional competence. Active and effective relationships between clients, practitioners, and educators is a further important element of professionalism.

All of the preceding suggests a complex set of problems and related opportunities available to the field of health administration, provided that the field can rise to the challenges which are presented. The normative definition which follows assumes that health administration can and must play an important role in the solution of problems of inequitable distribution and access, uneven quality, and inefficiency in the provision of health services. Through improved administration, the health of the total community can be promoted in a more equitable, comprehensive, high quality, and efficient manner. Accordingly, the following definition is offered:

> Health Administration is planning, organizing, directing, controlling, and coordinating the resources and procedures by which needs and demands for health and medical care and a healthful environment are fulfilled by the provision of specific services to individual clients, organizations, and communities.

The definition implies leadership in community policy decisions, as well as organization and management of resources gathered together in increasingly complex organizations. The administrative process must be carried out in socially responsible ways under conditions of continuous change and increasing uncertainly in the social, economic, political, technological, and professional environment.

Implications for practice

The definition suggests that health administrators can become a major force in solving many of the problems of our health care system. As mentioned previously, the problems to be solved are really only amenable to an administrative solution through improved planning, organization, financing, and performance evaluation of health and medical care. Some believe that the solution to all of these problems lies solely in provision of more professional manpower or better financing mechanisms. However, the complexities and pluralism of the delivery system as discussed in this paper suggest that provision of increased manpower or new financing mechanisms without attention to broader administrative matters may only aggravate the problems in our system.

In essence, some group within the system must pull it together. Administrators may be the logical group, provided that they can be both sensitive and pragmatic, responsive, and responsible. Anne Somers calls for positive leadership in the system with the following attributes: clear vision, intelligent strategy, adequate resources, determination, and courage.

Of primary importance, the definition suggests that extremely competent individuals will have to be attracted into the field if administrators are to "bite the bullet" and provide the leadership needed to bring about changes in the health and medical care system. Since formal educational programs serve a gate-keeping function for entry into the field, universities will need to attract students with a wide array of back-grounds, including minority groups and women, and with the native intelligence and personal attributes essential to future leadership roles.

The paper also suggests that educational programs must continue to pay attention to principles and techniques of modern management and systems theory, but must also prepare individuals who can operate effectively in the arena of public policy. Future administrators will need a solid understanding of health as health, rather than health as medical care (or sick care) planning and delivery.

Finally, close cooperation between educators and practicing administrators appears to be an essential ingredient. Researchers and educators must constantly question the way things are currently done and search for solutions to problems of the health services delivery system. Practitioners must participate by constantly reminding educators of the "art of the possible" and by providing the laboratory of real life experiences for students and faculty to utilize. Such a shared agenda will greatly facilitate the over-riding goal of providing leadership in response to complexity.

The growing need for motivated nurses

The nineteenth century angel of mercy has today been replaced by a seemingly less angelic and considerably more mercenary counterpart. With increased technical skill has come an apparent lessening of sensitivity to the sufferings of the patient. With demands for higher wages and better working conditions the modern Florence Nightingale is undoubtedly more efficient but somehow less comforting.

Sensitivity to the needs of the user

While this may seem a matter of minor moment to the hospital administrator, his management counterpart in other fields is showing growing concern with problems in motivation. He has already observed that with increased technical sophistication the product or service produced tends to become more important to the technician than the people using it. Pardonable pride in his technical accomplishments lessens his sensitivity to the needs of the user. This is particularly true when the product or service caters mainly to physical needs. Too often more subtle but equally real psychological needs are ignored or rationalized away.

In the admittedly difficult area of providing adequate nursing care for physically damaged and psychologically impaired patients, modern motivation theory gives rise to some interesting speculations and offers a strong possibility for marked improvement if seriously applied. To bring the topic into focus for the hospital administrator he must first be aware that one of his primary functions as a professional manager is the leadership and motivation of his subordinates. Its importance expressed in economic terms is most readily apparent in "strained" relationships with the patients, his customers. Time-consuming unreasonable demands and embarrassing complaints—all adding to operating costs—can be avoided if patients are properly motivated by the nursing staff. The nursing staff in turn must be motivated by their supervisors and the situations he encounters from his own particular point of view. The individual's perception of his environment is a conditioned reaction. It is conditioned by his own background and beliefs. Thus one employee may need careful supervision while another may function best with a minimum of supervision, When a supervisor stops by the desk of the first worker this may be interpreted as an expression of interest on the part of the supervisor. But the same act may be perceived by the second employee as unwarranted investigation or an expression of insufficient confidence in the ability of the worker to control his own performance.

Administrators must anticipate the reaction of employees to situations that arise. Only by an understanding of the individual his habits, expectations and beliefs can the administrator know what is needed to induce his spontaneous co-operation for the benefit of the organization.

The administrator must recognize the elements of satisfaction and dissatisfaction in the life of each member of the organization with whom he has direct relations. There is no short cut to sound human relations. The problems involved in meeting the needs of each employee are somewhat different from the problems presented by every other employee. Each man is unique, his situation differs in some respect for all others. Administrators must seek to understand the individual—his problems, his ambitions, the way he thinks and feels and why he has the attitudes he has. Patience and interest are required in order to determine the peculiarities of each member of the organization.

Inducing co-operation

It also must be recognized that expectations and interpretations are subject to change. They may be altered as a result of changes in other factors. As an employee becomes older he may become more interested in job security and retirement benefits. He may become somewhat less concerned with opportunities for advancement.

But the problem of inducing co-operation with the formal organization is even more complex. Administrators who are familiar with the sentiments expectations, and interpretations of individual employees may still fail to understand some of their behavior because of the influence of the informal organization.

Most formal organizational structures are comprised of smaller groups of employees who are in frequent contact with one another. Each individual will have frequent contacts with a relatively small number of people. These individuals often form identifiable groups. Their relations become standardized into certain patterns of acceptable behaviour; each person knows what is expected of him and what he can expect of others. These groups make effective technical cooperation possible. They increase stability, provide channels of communication, and routinize many relations. Individuals derive satisfaction and a sense of security from identifying themselves with groups of this informal type. In addition these groups have leadership positions that will be filled by one employee or another. They have certain relations with other groups, with supervisors and with the organization as a whole. The pattern of relations and the hierarchy of status positions that grow out of these natural groupings of people are called the "informal organization".

The informal organization influences the perception of the members of a formal organization. We are all influenced by social pressures. We try to meet the expectations of people with whom we are in frequent contact. We want their good will. As members of various groups and social organizations, we encounter group values, attitudes and sentiments that determine what is expected of the members of the group. We are subjected to considerable social pressure to conform to the group concept of acceptable behaviour.

The symbols of rank

The status hierarchy of the informal social organization is important to employees and is exemplified in every way possible. Each status position as associated with it certain customary symbols of rank. Everything in the work situation takes on a special meaning in terms of the social organization. Who gives directions to whom the relation of one employee's wages to those of other employees, the size of one, desk in relation to the desks of others, and every other variable becomes associated with certain positions in the informal social organization. Administrators who do not recognize this fact and treat objects and relations solely in terms of concepts of efficiency are likely to encounter difficulty in obtaining employee co-operation.

The informal social organizations of some employee groups serve to induce co-operation with administrators but other informal groups serve to limit co-operation. Therefore, the administrator must understand not only the individuals with whom he is in contact; he must also understand the informal groups into which they are organized. He must observe the attitudes and sentiments of these groups in order to be able to anticipate their reactions to various situations.

Once an informal pattern of relations and a hierarchy of status positions becomes established it tends to resist change. A change resulting from action taken by administrators may be interpreted as a threat to the stability or the continuation of the informal social organization. If it is, the change will be resisted and the members of the group will refuse to co-operate with their administrators.

Organisational treason

Changes in methods, organization or physical facilities that should produce substantial improvements in efficiency may result in drastically reduced efficiency if employees are suspicious or resentful of the change. The best systems cannot function properly if employees do not desire to see them succeed. The type of resistance, sometimes referred to as organizational treason must be expected unless support is obtained from employees in advance of any change.

The most effective way to obtain prior acceptance of change is to discuss with employees the problem that makes the change necessary. If employees are encouraged to participate in developing a solution, they will have an interest in seeing that the solution is effective. Under these conditions they will accept their responsibility to cooperate with other and they will strive to perform their assigned tasks in order to avoid a breakdown in the chain of interrelated functions. For example employees are always interested in receiving recognition as valuable members of an organization. If they are asked to participate in developing a cost-reduction program and their suggestions are seriously considered—they will support the final program of action. In this way the efficiency of the organization may be substantially increased.

7 Recruitment

New recruiting needs

Recruiting involves seeking and screening out qualified applicants and forming a pool from which job candidates are selected. As such, it is an integral part of human resources management. Health care organizations cannot function if they fail to attract quality applicants to fulfil their manpower requirements. This is particularly important in times of low unemployment when fewer people are available to work. Service organizations such as hospitals and clinics are labour intensive, hence vulnerable to shortages. Selection strategies, training programs, compensation systems, and career development programs can have only limited success if organizations cannot attract the work force they need.

There are few industries that employ personnel with such a wide range of expertise as health care. Physicians nurses technicians and semiskilled employees work interdependently to care for a patient. All these care givers and support staff are becoming increasingly dependent on administrators who know about the characteristics of the service area. ways to generate demand for service through marketing, and the intricacies of reimbursement. Several trends are making this already complex situation more complicated.

The health care industry is dramatically changing the mix of types of services offered as the burden of disease shifts. The United States is moving from an era of treating cases of acute, infectious diseases to managing patients with chronic diseases that periodically experience acute episodes. At the same time as third party payers have demanded reduction in the cost of care, user-friendly technologies have been perfected that allow a number of treatments to be given outside the hospital. The proliferation of clinical settings, including ambulatory surgery, skilled nursing and long-term care facilities, and home care, has created demands for types of personnel different from those found in a traditional community hospital. Furthermore, the linking of hospitals and alternative care facilities into multiunit diversified health care corporations has created a number of new management tasks, and hence manpower requirements. These positions in the corporate infrastructure, in headquarters and regional offices, for example, may entail planning productivity analysis or performance auditing. All the while, tertiary care facilities continue to need highly trained staff to work with increasingly complex technology and very sick patients.

Because of all these factors, the range and mix of skills required by health care personnel is expanding. This will complicate the work of a health care corporation's personnel department. For example, al large community hospital recently built a 12-bed hyperbaric chamber to treat burn and trauma patients but found few staff qualified to work there. The hospital had to either train nurses to work in those conditions or recruit deep-sea divers familiar with the hyperbaric technology and train them in nursing. The recruitment challenge created by this proliferation in requirements for skills and knowledge is further complicated by the location of the facilities. There are real differences in labour markets both between urban and rural settings, and among regions of the country Different recruiting strategies are necessary, then, for different types of staff and facilities of various types.

The discussion in this chapter can be simplified by dividing health care personnel into four categories.

Unskilled. Housekeeping, dietary, security

Technical workers. Nurses, technicians, therapists

Managers. CEO, department heads, controller, personnel director

Physicians. Contract. salaried, or merely medical staff members

This division will allow us to describe the common issues in recruiting as well as the distinctive problems that arise within each category. Although every issue will need to be addressed for each type of employee. The asterisks indicate that for specific employees there may be special problems that will affect strategies in terms of, for example the amount of planning needed, the time frame, or the geographic scope of the effort.

The recruitment process

The recruiting process consists of three basic steps: planning, implementation, and evaluation. To develop an effective recruiting program, six familiar questions must be answered: who, what, why, where, when, and how? The organization's plan explains why a position is required. An organization must then decide what types of positions must be filled and what types of people are needed to fill those positions who will recruit each job category, where candidates will be recruited from, and when the recruiting process must begin to ensure that the positions are filled by specified time. Once these decisions have been made, the plan can be implemented and a pool of candidates selected. To do this one needs to ask how the organization will attract qualified candidates and disqualify those who are clearly unsuitable. Then the program is evaluated, and the planning process beings once more.

Recruitment planning

Why? Demands for new strategies in human resources

Recruitment, selection and placement are closely linked functions of human resources management and can be leverage points for bringing about strategic change in an organization's goals or culture. In professionally dominated organizations. Practitioners have deeply ingrained work patterns as a result of their professional training and socialization. Recruiting and placing individuals who use different treatment protocols or have different work norms is one of the only ways to change these organizations.

Because of dramatic changes in the type of work in health care organizations, human resources planning and its recruitment component and to be closely tied to the overall planning process. Planning can be divided into three time frames.

- Strategic planning
- Tactical planning
- Operational planning

Plans focusing on each of these time frames should be updated periodically. Information generated by this ongoing planning process could change the focus or the scope of the recruiting effort.

Changes in an organization's strategic plans, such as diversification and vertical integration of services, could require dramatic changes in human resources, which in turn would call for new recruitment plans. For example, if a hospital starts an HMO, some physicians may need to be recruited. Their availability will need to be determined before the feasibility of this strategy can be assessed. Over a longer period, the case mix of an institution may change as a result of demographic changes in the service area from migration or from aging of the population. This could create incremental annual changes in staffing patterns, which would accumulate over time into significantly different staffing patterns, hence modified manpower requirements and recruiting needs.

At the tactical level, as hospitals "downsize" and shift more services into satellite offices internal recruiting strategies may need to change. There may be a number of employees who would rather transfer to a satellite clinic than be laid off. Testing and training may be necessary, though, to prepare these individuals for new jobs. Such changes would affect annual recruiting quotas and the size of the recruiting budget.

The reasons why an organization recruits different kinds of employees or physicians will continue to change. As these evolutionary changes occur an effective recruiting strategy will help to prevent.

- A shortage of labour
- Excessive use of overtime or excessive use of contract labour, such as pool nurses;
- Excesses of full-time equivalent (FTE) employees compared to some standard such as occupied beds or patient visits
- High training costs of new hires
- High turnover of new hires. suggesting a

mismatch between the applicants skills and actual job demands

- Physician or patient dissatisfaction with the staffs performance
- A poor image in the eyes of potential employees, suggesting that the organization has not been favourably represented in recruiting activities

What and when? Number and type of positions and timing of the search

Before any recruiting takes place, the management must determine how many positions need to be filled and what kinds. For physicians, this is a strategic decision under the purview of the board, medical staff, and top administrator that affects the service mix and in the long run the viability of the organization. Decisions about nurses, department managers and hourly workers have been the responsibility of the personnel function in the organization. In small organization these decisions are usually made on an ad hoc basis when line management informs personnel through employee requisition forms that position has been vacated or a new one created. However, large organizations, particularly organizations that need highly skilled employees must forecast their needs far in advance to ensure adequate staffing. Their need for employees in the future is determined by the strategic plans and the goals of the organization. Equal Employment Opportunity Commission (EEOC) regulations and affirmative action goals must also be taken into consideration. Organizations may be required to recruit specific minorities to redress past inequities. These needs must be compared to projected availability of human resources, and demands must be reconciled with supply. The results of this process will indicate to personnel staff the number and kinds of positions that need filled within a specified time frame .

The personnel staff must then determine how long it will take to successfully fill positions. Factors to be considered include the state of the economy, the technical and educational requirements of the positions to be filled and lead time for posting and advertising positions, and receiving and screening responses. Unskilled labor may be recruited in a week, but it may take 18 months to recruit a physician specialist. Nursing has presented a chronic recruiting problem. . For a variety of reasons relating to the unequal distribution of nurses, including external factors such as family obligations and undesirable working conditions in some facilities it will continue to be difficult to recruit nurses. Special efforts such as recruiting trips to professional conventions and job fairs will have to be planned far in advance.

The economy affects recruitment in several ways. First, the amount of unemployment will determine the size of the available labour pool This will affect various employee categories differently, but the amount of unemployment should be considered when timing and deciding the scope of a recruitment effort. Regional migration patterns that are economically motivated can also change the labour pool, hence recruitment plans. The technical and educational requirements of positions can tax the local labour pool. In these instances a wider search is needed, lengthening the amount of time required. Institutions have helped set up schools with specialized training programs for LPNs, RNs or various allied health positions to compensate for local labour shortages.

Decisions also have to be made on how many individuals to recruit for each job opening, since not all candidates will be acceptable and some acceptable candidates will decline job offers Historical data can be used to calculate yield ratios, comparing the number of candidates at each stage of the selection process to the number of candidates who make it to the next stage.

In the past physician recruitment either has not been done at all or has been done by the medical staff, but now, because of the strategic importance of recruiting the right kinds of subspecialists, hospital administration has become involved. An institution cannot implement a plan to diversify into certain services unless it has medical staff members willing to admit patients of those kinds. Also, as the number of staff model HMOs grows the number of salaried physicians will increase. Recruiting and selecting these physicians will become an increasingly important responsibility of management.

Deciding what types of physician are needed on the hospitals medical staff, hence, what types need to be recruited, is one area in which recruitment planning is inextricably tied to strategic and operational planning. This is always an executive function, but it is a support service that could be centralized in larger multiunit corporations.

Analyzing your medical staff for replacement purposes entails several steps.

- Categorize staff by specialty and prioritize based on importance to current plans.
- Note which physicians contribute more to the facility's profits. For cost-plus patients indicators include number of admissions, total patient days and number of ancillary procedures. As prospective payment becomes the norm, though more sophisticated measures will need to be developed. Someone who admits many patients for long stays that are not totally reimbursed could jeopardize the hospital's financial position.
- Note whether these physicians are located in parts of the service area where the facility capture a strong market share. Also note whether they are in areas where the hospital hopes to improve its position.
- The physicians ages should also be listed In this way one can predict when they will be reducing their practice or retiring. Knowing when medical staff in key subspecialties are retiring will indicate which type of staff to recruit and when.

Such an array quickly reveals any gaps in the current complement of physicians on the staff that may be due to the unavailability of certain key support staff. This would indicate further recruitment needs. Also future gaps can be identified as key physicians retire or reduce their practice. Any plans should also compare medical staff needs to the projected array of specialists at competing institutions A similar analysis can be done of the age structure of senior management personnel who are often costly to replace.

Efforts should soon be under way to replace some of the chief admitters at this hypothetical facility. National standards indicate shortages of chief admitters and several key admitters will be retiring soon. To recruit a physician and for him or her in turn to build up a practice takes several years so efforts should be started now. Possibly each of the senior key admitters could be encouraged to take on a partner who will eventually take over the practice.

Once a position as been targeted, it can take 18 months and cost up to $15.000 to recruit a physician. The board or medical staff may be reluctant to accelerate this process by incurring the cost of identifying the need and using a search firm. They should consider, however, what revenue could be generated if the needed physician were admitting 6 months sooner.

Who is responsible for recruiting

In most large organizations, recruiting is a function of the personnel department. Depending on the size of the department recruiting may be the responsibility of the director, a staffing unit, or a recruiting unit. The personnel staff recommends policy and strategy to top management seeks applicants for various sources, including the organization itself, screens applicants and form an applicant pool. When recruiting managers physicians or some technical staff line managers such as department heads or clinical chiefs, will take a more active role in the recruitment process. The complexity of federal regulations often requires that a personnel department members, such as an affirmative action officer, be in a position of functional authority over linestaff perhaps with authority to veto certain applicants or to reopen the process if correct procedures were not followed. This protects the organization from litigation form applicants who felt they were not treated fairly. A recruitment plan, then should state who should be involved and how each person will participate in the relevant phases of the process.

As care-giving facilities coalesce or merge into multiunit alliances and systems, many of the technical aspects of recruitment and other personnel functions are being centralized. Indeed recruiting on a wider geographic scope is espoused as one of the benefits of system affiliation. The recruitment functions that lend themselves to centralization include:

- Evaluating a facility's needs
- Developing a computerized skill bank that can be adapted for use by facilities

- Advertising and screening for needed technicians, nurses, managers, or physicians
- Tracking of laws and regulations, such as affirmative action guidelines
- Training facility staff to comply with regulations for example, when screening applicants
- Evaluating the cost effectiveness of facilities recruitment systems

Where recruiting sources and methods

Internal recruiting

One of the best courses of job applicants consists of the present employees of the organization. They are familiar with the culture and operations of the organization, and therefore, may be promoted or transferred into open positions with confidence that they will learn quickly. Also promotions are one of the best motivators organizations have at their disposal. Career opportunity at all hierarchical levels can account for the way people involve themselves in their work. Studies have shown that dramatic increases in opportunity can lead to increased career aspirations, higher work commitment, and a sense of organizational responsibility. Sometimes union contracts require management to consider internal candidates before looking outside the organization. The contract may also specify criteria to be used in developing an internal applicant pool.

There are several methods an organization can use to facilitate internal recruiting. First, job vacancies can be posted in public access areas and in company newsletters or bulletins. This gives the employees the opportunity to apply for positions that fit their needs. Second the organization can maintain a computerized skills inventory. This inventory may contain information on technical skills, supervisory experience, degrees obtained language skills, and even career aspirations. When a position becomes vacant or a new position is created, the organization will be able to quickly locate any potential candidates.

A third method of identical candidates for management slots is succession planning and the use of a replacement chart. It is a convenient way to show who is qualified to fill the different managerial positions in the facility. This approach is applicable only internally in large facilities but it is a useful way to keep track of managers working in various units in the system. By identifying transfers that best match the need of the positions with the career aspirations of the employees, there should be reduction in turnover as a result of increasing employees, satisfaction.

External recruiting

Although there are several advantages to recruiting internally, there are also some disadvantages. When organizations need to shift their direction quickly, bringing in new people with new ideas and new ways of doing things may be easier than trying to change all current employees. Also, the manpower an organization needs for the future may not always be available internally, This is particularly true in health care.

Organizations are expanding rapidly and technological developments constantly create a demand for new skills. Then, the organization must depend on the external labour market to fulfill its manpower requirements.

External recruitment becomes necessary as rapid diversification creates the need for new knowledge and skills not found in traditional health care setting. For example insurance sales persons are needed to market prepaid health service packages to employers. There has been some movement to recruit managers from outside industries just to infuse more business sense into hospitals or systems. It is not clear that this will be cost effective because of the unique characteristics of service industries in general and hospitals in particular.

The scope of the external search will depend on the types of position to be filled. The organization can generally rely on the local labor market fill lower level unskilled and semiskilled positions. Nurses or highly trained technicians may need to be recruited for a region-wide labor market. This may require strong affiliations with allied health schools in the area. Managers may need to be recruited nationally from health care and related industries. Physicians may need to be recruited nationally for certain subspecialties. Residency programs have traditionally been used to attract new physicians to an area in the hope that they will remain after completing the residency.

Whether the scope of the search is narrow or wide, an organization can utilize many different sources to attract and identify applicants. These include direct applications, employee medical staff, and other referrals; private and public employment agencies; executive search firms special events, and high schools, colleges, and universities. Television radio journal, and newspaper advertisements are the chief methods used to attract recruits.

Direct applications. If the organization has a good reputation and convenient location, direct applications may provide a large enough pool to fill all semiskilled and some technical positions at very little cost.

Employee, medical staff and other referrals. Many organizations rely on current employees to refer qualified applicants. Some organizations give cash bonuses to employees who encourage a friend or relative to apply for a position, if the applicant is hired. Additional cash bonuses may be paid if the referral remains employed by the organization for a specified time period.

The medical staff is probably not an adequate recruitment sources for physicians because of its geographic limits and the changing needs of the hospital. However the hospital exists in a complex network of relationships with suppliers sales people, licensing agents, and the like. These contacts are used to generate potential applicants. For example, sales representatives of suppliers to physicians, offices often can identify experienced but unhappy physicians.

Private and public employment agencies. Private employment agencies charge fees to perform many of the prescreening functions an organization would usually perform, such as finding qualified applicants, doing preliminary interviewing, and obtaining application blank information. Many of them specialize in, for example, nursing or technical personnel. The quality of private employment agencies varies tremendously, so the organization may have to do some searching before finding one that adequately meets its needs.

Public employment agencies are operated by the states under the auspices of the US Training and Employment Service. All men and women who collect unemployment insurance are required to use this service which is free to both seekers and organizations Public employment agencies now utilize computer systems to match applicants with jobs Few organizations. However, take advantage of this service, since employers complain that the referrals often are poorly qualified and not always interested in accepting employment.

Executive search firms. These highly specialized private employment agencies usually seek candidates currently earning $40,000 or more. They are more expensive and more aggressive than other private agencies, generally charging half an executive's annual salary as a fee. Whereas most private employment agencies rely on candidates who are actively looking for a position, executive search firms often called "head hunters" will approach highly qualified professionals who are currently employed and had not been looking. Industry norms forbid hospitals to recruit employees directly from one another. Thus headhunters may serve a useful purpose by broadening the pool of applicants for organizations that need upper level executives.

Care should be taken however to contract with a reputable firm. Table lists some characteristics that distinguish reputable from disreputable executive search firms.

Special events. Job fairs and meetings of professional societies provided convenient setting for an organization's recruiter to meet with potential employees or search firms job fairs are often regional events in which employers in certain industries can met with interested applicants and promote their organisations job openings.

High schools, colleges and universities. Educational institutions are good sources of applicants for positions that require very little experiences. High school and vocational schools are good applicant sources for low skilled and trade positions. In some communities businesses develop and partially fund training programs in conjunction with educational institutions. This arrangement provides the businesses with a readily available pool of qualified applicants.

Nursing schools have often been developed by larger hospitals. The professionalisation of the field, with a concomitant raising of educational requirements has forced many of the schools not associated with colleges or universities to close in recent years. There continues to be a shortage of specialized nurses, in operating rooms and intensive care units for example, suggesting a need for more continuing education programs.

Colleges and universities are good applicant sources for nursing and managerial positions as well as physicians. Many universities now have specialized programs in health care administration. The Association of University Programs in Health Administration publishes a directory of all member graduate and under graduate health administration programs in the United States and Canada these require students to participate in either summer internships or longer residencies before graduating. Also there are a growing number of competitive fellowships being offered. These usually require a 2-year commitment and often are based in the corporate offices of multiunit systems.

Finally, hospital affiliation with medical schools in order to employ residents has long been a means of recruiting physicians in local communities. Search firms recruit directly at medical schools or residency sites.

Other than working with the sources mentioned above, the major method of recruiting is through advertising.

Advertisements. Organizations can advertise position openings in newspaper and journals on television and radio, and on even billboards.

Organizations often consult with advertising agencies to determine the most effective medium and content of a recruitment campaign recruitment campaign.

Advertisement should convey the qualifications and major responsibilities of the position as well as the working conditions. If the organization is a government contractor, the advertisement must indicate that the organization is an equal opportunity employer. An advertisement implying that a candidate of a particular race, sex, religion age, and/or nationality is preferred over others is illegal, unless the organization can prove that these characteristics are bona fide occupational requirements. According to Section 703(e) of Title VII of the Civil Rights Act of 1964, an organization may discriminate on the basis of race, sex, religion, age, or national origin if the attribute is a bona fide occupational qualification (BFOQ), reasonably necessary to the normal operation of that particular business or enterprise.

In developing an advertising campaign, an organization must also take into consideration the message it wants to convey to the public and the audience it wants to target. Lower level, unskilled and semiskilled workers can best be reached through want ads in local newspapers or radio advertisements. Professional and technical workers are more likely to respond to advertisements in trade publications. Placing advertisements in publications of these types is particularly worth while if the level of expertise required for the position is not available through the local labour market. Trade and professional journals are distributed nationally and sometimes internationally, so they reach a wider and more specialized audience. A good list of journals and mailing lists for advertising job openings to the nursing labour market is given by Filoromo and Ziff.

8 Behavioural System

Professionals in health services organisations

One of the greatest problems facing managers of health services organisations is associated with the complexity of having many different occupations and occupational groupings represented in the same institutional structure. For example, a mental health clinic may employ psychologists, psychiatrists, social workers, psychiatric technicians, and counsellors, to name a few. Health maintenance organisations may employ nurses, physicians, health educators, physicians, assistants, nurse practitioners, and support personnel. Large group practices may employ many of the professionals used in health maintenance organisations, plus attorneys and certified public accountants. All these health services organisations may also have affiliations with professional consultants who are not salaried by the organisations. These consultants may receive their compensation as fee for service, but their influence on the organisation and its other employees may be very significant: that is, considerably less tenuous than the term "consultant" implies.

A question confronting the managers of health services organisations is the issue of how to manage, control, motivate, and reward the professionals who have strong ties with the organisation as well as those who are less firmly connected. This section presents the concepts of professionals in organisations and some of the factors that appear to affect the behaviour of professional within the organisation.

Health services organisations require the services of professionals of many types. Defining which individuals are classified as professionals sometimes causes difficulties for managers because it seems as if many occupations groups are asking managers and society in general to treat them as professional. In fact, these definitional difficulties have been recognized by theorists for decades and have resulted in many articles. One of the best known, entitled "The professionalization of everyone?", presents the quandary most thoroughly.

In health services organisations, one would expect to find a variety of occupations represented. Many of these occupations have experienced the natural evolution toward professionalism. Members have formed professional associations, instituted codes of ethics, encouraged more rigorous credentialing and licensing of practitioners, and urged an increase in educational requirements. The health services manager must ascertain how different and how similar are these 'new' professionals from the occupations that have been considered historically to be professions. Do they require or expect autonomy as a prerequisite for satisfaction with the work environment? Do they experience conditional loyalty to the organisation? Will there be a difference between the expectations instilled in the "new" professional during training and the conditions and expectations of the employing organisation? How does the manager identify and define the professional occupations?

Definition of professional

Historically, the professions were defined as the ministry, law, and sometimes medicine. As educational levels increased in the United States, and as our economy moved away from an industrial base toward being service based, more and more groups of highly trained individuals who called themselves professionals emerged in our society.

On what basis does an occupation become designated a "profession"? It is generally accepted that professionals are highly trained in an area of expertise and are certified by some institutions. As a result, they possess specialized knowledge and may be considered experts in their fields. They have a commitment, considered to be enduring, to their professions. Also, many professionals feel that they are dealing with areas of social or universal concern, and they are seen as providing a service.

Professionals desire autonomy in their work environment and many groups of professionals believe that only their peers are qualified to judge their work. Because of their specialized training, professionals expect to establish their standards and codes of ethics. Thus, autonomy and independence are conditions that help differentiate professionals from other employees in organisations.

Because of tho proliferation of groups calling themselves professional, there has been an effort to find a general definition or common denominator describing all professions. Such definitions have ultimately emphasized autonomous expertise, the service orientation ideal, and a high level of technical training. The amount of autonomy the health professional is allowed to exercise becomes a very real indicator of a profession. Thus, physicians have historically been thought to belong to a profession as defined here, since they have had the most autonomy in healthy care settings. Members of other health related occupations also experience autonomy within the confines of their job responsibilities and would qualify as professionals

Individuals who consider themselves to belong to professional occupations in health organisations can be divided into four groups. Each group brings its own orientations, its own set of priorities, and its own goals, which may conflict with those of other professionals. One group consists of nurses and allied health workers. Another group consists of physicians. A third group consists of technicians. The final group consists of managerial personnel. There is some debate concerning whether all four groups possess all the attributes associated with professions. Yet it is worthy of note that each of these groups in one way or another, identifies itself as a professions. The remarks in the section that follows apply to professionals and professional behaviour in varying degrees, depending on how closely the individuals and occupations are aligned with the definitions of a profession.

Conflict for professionals

Professionals may experience conflict working within a bureaucracy because the profession and the bureaucracy are based on fundamentally different principles of organisation. In a bureaucracy, for example, certain conditions exist such as a hierarchical structure and delineated formal procedures, with rules and controls. Specialization of labor, with few workers trained or hired to produce the entire product, is another feature of many bureaucracies. Professional behaviour, however, is centered on commitment to autonomy and peer review. The conflict arises when the professional is employed by the bureaucratic organisation, and the professional's requirement for autonomy is incongruent with the bureaucracy's need for structure and control.

There is some indication that this conflict is not inevitable: professional attitudes and commitment to a bureaucratic organisation are not necessarily incompatible. Health care workers such as nurses or research scientists may find that the bureaucracy supports their professional goals by supplying them with a structure that facilitates their work. In fact, there is slight evidence that physicians and their feelings of autonomy can be affected positively by bureaucracies, but researchers are going to have to investigate this condition more thoroughly in health services organisations.

Conditional loyalty

The professional's behaviour within the organisation may be best understood via the concept of conditional loyalty, which occurs because the professional identifies first with his or her profession and then with the work organisation. This strong form of identification is established and fostered when the professionals receive their training and is perpetuated through professional groups and associations in which they maintain membership. Through the extensive, and often lengthy, training professionals receive, they develop a "professional" self image: They value their skills highly and are more concerned with their reputations among their peers than with pleasing organisational superiors: they view the organisation and its administrators as facilitators, and their loyalty to the organisation may be conditional upon their evaluation of the adequacy of the organisation's facilities and programs relative to others of which they are aware.

Other types of employee may also experience a conditional loyalty to the organisation, especially part time employees. This tendency is especially important for health services organisations that employ or affiliate with individuals on a quasi-contractual basis—for example agency nurses who are available for temporary duty during periods of peak demand, physicians who come as consultants, or employees of a contracted housekeeping service. Such persons may enter the organisation with fewer and different expectations concerning the role the organisation will assume in their lives as contrasted with the full-time salaried employee. Employees expectations of the organisation are related to their levels of commitment and motivation.

The example that follows illustrates the type of conflict that occurs among professionals health services in organisations.

Ms. Carter, director of nursing at General Hospital, a 140-bed community hospital, is disturbed that the administration has vetoed the nursing department's equipment request for a microprocessor for use in patient care planning. In addition, the cardiology medical staff has just received a denial of a $5000 request for new equipment. Both the nurses and the cardiologists feel that the denials were arbitrary and that their needs were not evaluated fairly. They have complained formally to Ms Carter and to the chief of the medical staff, Dr. Johnson, who have asked that the senior administrator, Ms. Bells, consider their appeal. The central argument is that the organisation's failure to assign priorities in the allocation of the hospital's financial resources in improper: "Whenever the nursing or medical staff requests equipment, we have to justify and rejustify our needs, but when the administration wants to renovate their offices, the money is spent without any input from us. What's the difference? Who approves their justification? Do they even have to provide a justification? Patient care needs should be met first. "Mr. Bells responds by saying that he too is a professional who knows what is best for the organisation and that he takes everybody's needs into account when he makes allocation decisions.

Increasing conflict

As more and more health services organisations are pressured to be efficient producers of quality health care, and especially in this era of changing reimbursement systems, conflict between health care professionals and administrators is increasing in some environments. One of the primary reasons for the increase in conflict is the perception that what is in the best interest of the patient will become secondary to the goal of efficient delivery of that care. This conflict is demonstrated most dramatically by changes occurring to professionals such as physicians. Some physicians believe that they have lost control of their profession. More and more physicians are working on salary rather than fee for service, and they are beginning to feel like "hired hands." They are attacked in editorials in local newspapers, and in national publications such as the Wall Street Journal as being unresponsive to changes occurring in the delivery of health care. They feel as if they have fallen victim to a reimbursement system and to third party payers who are controlling the future of medicine rather than being allowed to concentrate on what is best for the patient. Hospitals expanding their outpatient clinics are perceived to be in direct competition with physicians: alternative delivery systems are affecting their patient mix as well as their incomes;relative value scales bring economic uncertainty.

Health professionals are feeling forms of attack in addition to increasing competition and changing reimbursement systems. Changing liability and malpractice laws, changing Joint Commission on the Accreditation of Hospitals requirements, changing regulations encouraging more review of medical decisions, and greater numbers of professionals and occupations, as well as a better educated society questioning their decisions and judgment, are all contributing to a significantly changed environment for health professionals.

Professionals may see their role in the health care organisations in terms completely different from those used by organisational management. The professional may view himself or herself as a scientist working for a patron, whereas the organisation sees the relationship in terms of client professional, or even employer employee. This role ambiguity undoubtedly will contribute to dissatisfaction or decreased levels of organisational commitment.

Health professionals may complain about administrator's interference in clinical decision making and administrator's contributing to inefficiencies in the delivery of health care. They may perceive that they are losing their professional independence. On the other hand, health professionals may find that the accomplishment of their professional goals is facilitated by the marketing and management support provided by these very administrators. If administrators are assisting the clinician in the acquisition of needed or desired resources, a form of team building between the two groups may occur. Conditional loyalty to the health services organisation may become contingent on the provision by the organisation of needed support to the physician or clinician.

Organisations that have interactions with health professionals in this rapidly changing environment are using various methods to alleviate this conflict. Some of the new forms of organisational design are presented next.

Organisational forms used by health professionals

The relationship between health services providers and health services organisations has been formalized in several ways, which were described by Scott in 1982.

Autonomous structure

The institution may delegate to the professional group the responsibility for setting goals and standards, and for seeing that the standards are maintained. This type of arrangement is justified because of the complexity and uncertainty involved in the work performed, conditions especially applicable in health services organisations. Many professionals, because of their training, ascribe to the system of peer review as a form of control and review of their performance. Only professional colleagues are believed to possess the specialized training and experience that would permit valid evaluations of performance. The administrations does not have control over the quality or type of professional practice occurring in the health care organisation.

Many general hospitals have an autonomous form of organisation: that is, the governing board has delegated the legal responsibility for the care of patients to the medical staff. The medical staff in organisations of this type has organized formally to determine the physicians who will be granted admitting privileges. The degree of organisation of the medical staff varies with the individual health organisations. Some hospitals, for example, have a medical staff that operates as a very organized collective unit. Others have a staff comprised of a loosely connected group of individuals who do not view themselves as part of a group or a formal structure.

Various control arrangements in addition to peer review exist in organisations with this type of professional structure. The JCAH has described minimal credentialing requirements for medical staff and various committees involving physicians as a requirement of the health services organisation. Federal regulations associated with reimbursement have also established controls, such as the Peer Review Organisation, which reviews elective Medicare hospital admissions on a prospective basis. This type of preadmission review is being required by other third-party vendors, such as commercial insurance carriers, and by health maintenance organisations, in an attempt to encourage more appropriate inpatient utilization. The PRO constitutes a significant control on physicians, and physicians have reorganized some of their administrative and clinical procedures in response to the introduction of this institution.

Administrative dominance of health professional

In a second kind of organisational form, professionals in health organisations do not have the kind of autonomy described previously and are subjected to regular supervision and instruction. In most health service organisations, nurses are a part of this administrative dominance type of structure. Also included are groups such as physical therapists and medical technologists. The case study entitled "Professionals at West End Hospital" demonstrates this type of organisational form.

Professional at West End Hospital

> The Department of Health Services Research at West End Hospital is composed of highly educated and highly trained professionals whose goal is to provide many forms of biostatistical information to various areas of the hospital. Within this department is the Cardiac Disease Registry, a group of technical employees who gather data on all the cardiac patients in the hospital.

Much of the work of the registry was done by registered records administrators who possessed bachelor's degrees and were trained to abstract clinical information from medical records. They were paid relatively little for doing highly technical but routine and tedious work. The RRAs were supposed to be on an equal administrative level with holders of master's and doctoral degrees, but these professionals had difficulty imagining that anyone less highly trained and educated than themselves might perform research functions.

As time progressed other professionals, accredited records technicians, were added to the Cardiac Disease Registry to perform follow up functions. This information was added to the basic data base to give a full and complete picture of the cardiac patients and what happened to them over time.

All these factors began to take a toll on the registry members and one by one as professional openings with a new outlook and challenge as well as better compensation came along, the RRAs left the registry. Not unexpectedly word of the registry's situation spread, and it became difficult to recruit new RRAs for the positions that were available.

As a part of a hospital-wide program, the

job descriptions for these positions were reevaluated and rewritten for the registry personnel. After consideration of the skills necessary to perform the registry functions a new job description was written for a technician rather than a trained, degreed professional.

The job analysts determined that trained professional skills were not needed to perform chart abstracting. The job actually required knowledge of the medical record order and catheterization report format and familiarity with the variables to be abstracted from both these sources. The job itself was fairly routine and repetitious and the skills could be learned on the job by performing the abstracting duties. A general knowledge of medical terminology was an advantage but this could be assimilated over time by working with the medical records and catheterization reports. Clinical skills required were also minimal because routine information was given in the catheterization report format of history, physical and laboratory values anatomy procedures, findings and diagnosis on each patient. The single most difficult part of the abstracting after familiarity with the variables was acquired was interpreting the physician's catheterization report. This too was expected to become less difficult in time and after the analyst came to know each physician's style of presenting information.

The follow-up positions in the registry involved slightly different skills but again it was decided that professional skills were not necessary. Basically the job was to update the data base using income information from follow up questionnaires. These skills could again be mastered over time and on the job.

From both these job analyses new job descriptions were complied that became almost generic. The job descriptions followed the basic format of listing job title, job summary and duties and responsibilities in the job description portion and enumerating employee qualifications to perform the job satisfactorily in the job specification portion.

Once selected and hired new registry employees were trained by a senior member of the registry unit. The length of time for training varied with the individual but the goal was to enable the new employees to achieve productivity standards outlined in the performance appraisal for the position.

A productivity profile was kept on each abstract assistant. Although it is somewhat difficult to quantify the work of the abstract assistants and impossible to do so for the follow up assistants, some figures of productivity are necessary for such a large group of employees to justify their existence to administration and to continue to be budgeted.

The performance of each employee is appraised annually to provide information needed for determining whether individual work results are consistent with expectation and for identifying high marginal and unsatisfactory performance. Information on compensation determination is also received as well as feedback for both employee and supervisor.

At one time a type of management by objectives was accomplished by these performance appraisals in that both employee and supervisor would independently list goals to be accomplished within a time frame chosen by the employee. These objectives were discussed privately and a common list for each employee was compiled through the joint efforts of employee and supervisor. Now however the supervisor lists objectives and deadlines for each employee and the list is conveyed to the employee at the time of evaluation.

The retention of registry analysts once trained is affected by several factors both positive and negative. The negative factors can be summed up under the overall topic of motivation. These employees have lower than expected motivation levels because of perceived inquiry in status with their departmental coworkers, lack of opportunity for advancement because of the emphasis on degrees in the other units of the department and poor communication associated with relations with the other members of the department as well as unclear lines of responsibility and accountability.

The positive factors almost outweigh the negative and make retention of employees possible. Benefits within the organisation are fair, but possibly the department's best benefit is its "flex time" policy. This is appealing to the personnel presently in the registry, many of whom are mothers of young children. Because time schedules are somewhat flexible and time can be made up within a pay period, loss of pay and attendance holidays because of children's illnesses and so on is not a threat.

The registry positions also offer an entry into the organisation and can help individuals to be aware of other hospital positions and possible advancement.

And how have the registry personnel

achieved at least the basic esteem level of Maslow's hierarchy? Over time they have gained acceptance for their skills within the department through recognition of what their job involves and what a valuable source of information their data base is. For example, a recent newspaper article was able to quote mortality figures for cardiac patients using the data base. Also university physicians are now using the data base for research and publication. Articles and presentations of national distribution have come from this large data base.

The merging of two different types of personnel both of whom consider themselves to be professional has been a challenge for the health service research department of West End Hospital Understanding professional behaviour and factors influencing the motivation of these employees has helped in providing an environment conducive to the retention of these employees.

In some environments physicians are coming more and more under the administrative dominance type of organisation because of the changes that are occurring rapidly in health care and because of the new organisational forms that are emerging. There are many reasons for these changes. The need for additional coordination of the many specialized activities associated with patient care has become more apparent. Changing reimbursement mechanisms are putting institutions more at risk financially because of the activities of the professionals associated with those institutions. Physicians are increasingly dependent on hospitals or other institutions to provide their practice environment, and many are becoming salaried by these institutions.

The professionals working in this type of organisation are not organized separately into an autonomous unit. There is much more overlapping of administrative and professional actions. However an individual professional still has considerable discretion over clinical decision making and tasks. Administrators, many of them clinical professionals themselves coordinate the activities of these individuals. This form of organisation is seen in some academic medical centers and in the Veterans Administration health units. Teams are used frequently for the provision of patient care, forming a type of product line management focus, as is common in industrial organisations.

What form is the most appropriate for the resolution of conflict described previously? There is no general agreement. However the section that follows describes one approach that allows for the special requirements of professionals.

Resolution of conflict

Some health services organisations are attempting to resolve the conflict occurring when professionals work in bureaucracies. They are establishing coequal professional groupings in which the medical staff hierarchy and the administrative hierarchy are roughly equal in power and importance, and are interdependent. Communication vehicles and participation in decision making contribute to this perception of equality. Under this form, health professionals are concerned with the delivery of patient care to individual patients, and administrators are concerned with the larger issues of patient care, the delivery of care to groups of patients. There is no longer the artificial and increasingly inefficient distinction of having patient care issues decided by the medical staff, and support and maintenance issues by the administrators.

Both groups, the health professionals and the administrators need to be kept informed of the other group, concerns. For example, when the hospital must choose between allowing a nonpaying nonemergency patient to be admitted and reducing the amount of care provided to paying patients in a systematic manner, the health professionals must be kept informed of the nature and complexity of the dilemma faced by the administrators.

9 The History of Hospital and Human Resources Information Systems

The need for collection ·analysis, and management use of human resources information has outpaced the development of human resources information systems in health care institutions. Even hospital information systems which have made significant progress over the past two decades continue to evolve 8-12 years behind other industries. Increases are largely attributed to the expanding functions of information systems especially in patient care and strategic management application—two areas experiencing pressure for management accountability. To further enhance this evolution, technological developments have greatly improved the ability of managers to have direct access to multiple data bases, including human resources variables. For the most part, however, there remains much scope for improvement and managers remain frustrated by the lack of accessibility to human resources information.

The use of information systems in hospitals began during the 1960s and has evolved in five stages.

Stage 1. Early hospital information systems had traditional module capabilities to process business office paperwork such as patient billing, accounts receivable, payroll, and general ledger. Information systems were not used in personnel departments. In other industries large organizations began installation of HRIS in the 1960s.

Stage 2. By the 1970s about a third of community hospitals had begun to use computers. Limited data collection systems were developed, which incorporated the capabilities of financial information systems. In the early 1970s many larger hospitals implemented computer systems for productivity planning, and analysis.

By the early 1970s commercial software products became available that offered multifunctional capability—a single system to serve the needs of all human resources activities. By the late 1970s-most organizations in other industries had begun to install HRIS. One important impetus for the growth of human resources information systems in hospitals during this period was the increased number of employee protection laws, which grew out of the social and legislative environment of the 1960s and 1970s. These acts called for complex personnel reporting systems to state and federal governments and led to automated data bases on recruitment placement transfer and promotion history, job description performance review, and vested and accrued benefits.

Stage 3. During the 1970s there was limited development of medical information systems. Systems were implemented to meet the operational needs of hospitals: scheduling, reporting and management of the work load. Advances were made in laboratory and radiology reporting pharmacy systems, scheduling of systems or operating rooms, and systems for admitting and locating patients. After the 1970s, a central feature of the progress of computer information services was the automation of medical records and the development of intelligent work stations serving integrated systems. Human resources information remained isolated in the personnel department When analysis occurred, data had to be retrieved from multiple independent sources. Output was independent from the rest of the information system. Interface between data bases remained a low priority.

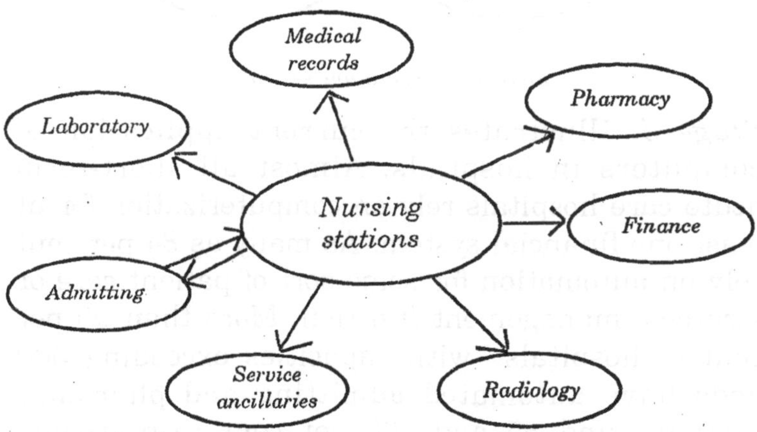

Data collection systems

Stage 4. Developing hospital information systems to support day-to-day operations was the focus of the 1980s The increasing demand for improved employee benefits and financial security was a major contributory factor in the development of HRIS during this period period. Benefit plans in particular became increasingly complex. Necessitating automated record keeping.

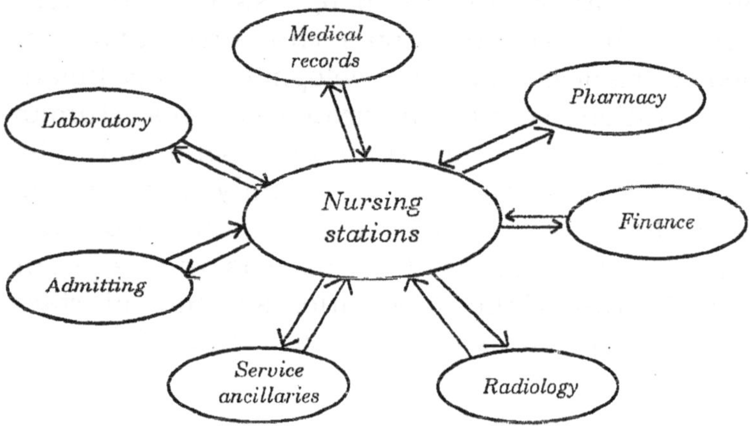

Medical information systems

Stage 5. Illustrates the current application of computers in hospitals. Almost all short-term acute care hospitals rely on computerization for at least one financial system. As many as 84 per cent rely on automation for some sort of patient care or strategic management function. More than 90 per cent of hospitals with capacities exceeding 500 beds have automated admitting and pharmacy systems, and 85 and 68 per cent respectively, have laboratory systems and nursing stations automated.

The trend in health care information systems is increasingly toward the development of integrated hospital information systems. Hospital computer systems are now being programmed for interrelating information from different data bases with computer and telecommunication systems physically linked into a common network. Few organizations in health care have, however, achieved the goal of an integrated approach to information gathering and communication. Few attempt to coordinate software acquisition or to force data base compatibility. It is not uncommon to find large organizations in which all the departments use different vendors. One reason may be that no single vendor is currently able to handle most needs of a complex health care system. The explosion in telecommunications development is rapidly helping to alleviate data incompatibility problems. The major problem in the future will be "data overload" as a result of the lack of careful and selective planning about what information to collect and analyze. Most institutions today face inadequate information retrieval and modelling capability and have isolated systems that cannot communicate with corporate systems. For example, few organisations have the capacity to provide employee skill information throughout the institution for purposes of manpower planning, recruitment, or hiring.

Most human resources information systems continue to be used for record retention and report generation. Murdich and Schuster found that employee identification, payroll, equal employment opportunity compliance data, and compensation functions are the most widely computerized human resources functions. Little or no forecasting modelling, or trend analysis is applied to these systems. These weaknesses critically hinder an institution's ability to compete.

Other trends in the evolution of automated information systems in health care facilities include the following.

1. Increased budgets for internal MIS
2. Increased capacity and reliability
3. Improvement in business-oriented software
4. Growth in communications;
5. Microcomputer technology providing distributed processing

Traditionally, however, hospital personnel department functioned solely for operational levels of management providing support for such activities as wage and salary administration, benefit administration, recruitment, and government reporting. Record keeping was minimal and was applied directly to these areas of operations. Personnel departments were not perceived as having role in organizational planning or decision making. Information available in the personnel department-often collected manuals—was typically not used by management.

In the 1970, new technologies in information systems allowed for automation of personnel data and coordination of previously separated data bases. Personnel departments began to automate operational procedures, saving staff time for other activities. Computerized reporting provided the capability to offer data on staff activities and trends to department heads and management.

This capability has paralleled a growing demand for information about the human resource in health institutions. As they evolve from social based organizations to competitors in the world of big business, most health institutions are struggling to maintain or expand their position in the marketplace. With the current environment of competitive pricing and heavy regulation, positioning in the market place is not as stable as in the past but is open to challenge from resourceful and imaginative organizations.

Strategies for coping with this environment vary but generally include some attempt to reduce costs without compromising the quality of care to patients. Whatever their strategy managers must answer two key questions:

Are the institution's costs competitive?

How can the quality of service provided be maintained?

Answers to these key business problems contain essential human resources elements that must be addressed as part of the organizational strategy. Furthermore, all decisions made or actions taken will affect the nature of the relationship between the organization and its employees.

Consider a business strategy to compete by becoming a low-cost producer of health care services. The internal plan may be to increase productivity and reduce staff levels while making an effort to improve performance. Managers would need to scrutinize labor force levels, productivity, skills, and employee commitment. Alternatively, a new technology introduced into a hospital, a merger between facilities or the approval of new services would also involve important human resources decisions. These decisions and the manner in which they are implemented can reinforce or undermine the effective use of personnel.

In this environment and given the greater availability of information technology, human resources departments will increasingly play an active role in providing information and analytical skills to assist management in achieving its strategic objectives.

This broadened role of HRM is reflected in the use of information about human resources that no longer will be viewed as a separate function unique to the personnel department but will contribute to many different departments and levels of the organization. Consider a typical personnel data bases of the past, which consisted only of a payroll system that produced paychecks and labour reports. Today the HRIS would provide added management support by consolidating several personnel variables into a forecast of work loads staffing and scheduling. Or, consider the role of employee skill inventories which has broadened to include use in matching applicants with jobs, planning career development with employees performing succession planning and making manpower projections. Or, consider employee files, which contain names of supervisors and their subordinates. This listing, probably not used in the past, is increasingly used for scheduling training for supervisors, contacting supervisors about training opportunities for subordinates, tracking the performance appraisal process, or mailing, notices about policy or procedural changes. These examples point out that human resources data gathered for one purpose increasingly serve a number of purposes and are accessed throughout the organization.

A model of human resources information systems

So far we have emphasized the application of human resources information systems for planning the business strategy of the organization. Our perspective has been that of the planner or top manager whose decisions may affect the overall organization. In this section we broaden the approach to provide model for an HRIS that reaches other management levels.

Understanding the roles HRIS can play throughout the organization requires taking systems perspective of health care institution. Systems theory provides a view of the health organization as a system made up of separate but united subsystems which work together to serve the goal of the total system. In taking this view we see how information systems can become an important tool for supporting individual care delivery subsystems, while also integrating these subsystems for purposes of corporate policy. The rapid development of complex health systems and diversification of health structures has forced health care managers to look at their organization as subsystems of larger systems rather than as is isolated units with discrete structures and information needs.

A vertically integrated system may be composed of heterogeneous organizations such as acute care hospitals outpatient units, long term care units, and other chronic care units. Each contains subsystems that could be further divided into a series of smaller subsystems. For example the auto care hospital will contain a patient care subsystem that is composed of smaller subsystems. The entire network of systems and subsystems works synergistically in a structured way to compromise that total multi-institutional system.

10 Management in Human Service Organisations

Any individual performing clinical tasks in human services, such as a social caseworker a psychiatrist or a counsellor approaches his or her client or patient with some kind of framework in mind. The clinician's framework contains a number of indicants and variables that reveal certain dynamics providing the clinician with an analysis of a given situation. This framework is the basis on which a clinician understands client problems and recognizes certain behavioural patterns or syndromes concerning individual functioning; it represents the foundation on which the clinician devises appropriate interventions leading to an alleviation of the problem. Some concept of optimal functioning as well as an organized notion of the variety of possible interventions, is therefore necessary. The clinician is conscious of this framework or key aspects of it, as he or she engages in clinical tasks. A new or inexperienced clinician may apply frame-work in a relatively structured and mechanistic manner, but with experience, the use of such a framework typically becomes more 'natural' and more easily applied.

The preceding chapters presented a similar kind of framework for the human service manager. This framework provides indicants and variables that the practitioner must observe, understand and assess. The framework indicates how these factors merge to form dynamics that are both functional and dysfunctional to service effectiveness. Like the clinician the manager uses the framework to shape his or her thinking about an organisation, asseses established pattern of functioning that either enhance or detract service delivery from and evoke appropriate interventions.

In a human service organisation, as in all organisations, there are individuals who function in staff or line positions. Their primary task in a human service organisation consists of activities other than providing direct service to clients or patients. The number of organisational members engaged in these processes varies greatly with the human service organisation in question. In a small agency the executive director a few immediate staff and a small number of supervisors may perform all the functions of management. In a large organisation, such as a state hospital, the people performing these functions may number several hundred.

In this chapter we consider the process of management. First we define service and maintenance management and address their relationship. We then examine the strategies of management that conclude with a discussion of managerial style.

Definitions of management: Service management and maintenance management

Following the framework, it is important to differentiate service management from maintenance management; to distinguish between managerial activities that actually help to enhance service to clients from those activities which serve to maintain the organisation and help ensure its survival. It is service management and maintenance management which combine to form the managerial process in human service Organisations. This process can be termed human service management.

Service management

In leading a human service organisation to a pattern of most effective service, management as concerned with the highest possible quality of service resources as input, and optimization of these resources in the throughput. In general, this requires the recruitment and development of human technology and technological ability, the pursuit of congruent decision-making, adherence to official goals, and authority based on professional ability in the internal functioning of an organisation. It means, as well, the careful guiding of factors external to an organisation that influence service outcome, as well as procedures internal to the organisation that may influence the patterns of service effectiveness. In short, service management represents a series of tasks in a human service organisation that carry the responsibility for the overall quality of the organisation, service product Service management needs to be based on a careful analysis of how organisational functioning affect, the quality of service provided by the organisation. In this way service management can ensure increased effectiveness in human service Organisations leading to the strengthening of the social welfare institution.

Maintenance management

Although as noted that service resources distinguish human service organisations from other formal organisations, these resources are not the sole input. All organisations require maintenance resources in order to function such as equipment, materials for upkeep, physical plant, support staff, funding and so on. Maintenance management is primarily concerned with the procuring, processing and allocating of maintenance resources and material and with the operation of the organisation in terms of the efficient integration of its components which in include the reduction for organisational conflict and the achievement of organisational equilibrium and consensus. Maintenance management is concerned then with producing a "well-run" organisation. It is concerned with such tasks as the standardization, coordination, and general execution of the rules, regulations, and procedures of an organisation. Therefore maintenance management is directed toward efficiency in the use of resources and with survival rather than with the effectiveness of service. Of course a smoothly operating organisation which is physically responsible and accountable and whose components adhere to procedures conserve resources and demonstrate consensus may be a well-run organisation form a maintenance perspective but may still deliver a vastly inferior service product. By the same token however, the importance of successful performance of maintenance management in human service organisations cannot be overemphasized. This is particularly true in an era characterized by the need on the part of human service organisations cannot be overemphasized to demonstrate efficiency and accountability. The cry of "mismanagement" has been constant one and has often been made with some justification. Both human service organisations and the overall social welfare institution are very much dependent on the successful execution of maintenance management, without it, the service product of the Organisation will ultimately suffer.

The relationship between service and maintenance management

A major problem of balance can often lie between maintenance and service management. This relationship can affect the functioning of the organisation and its service product. As previously mentioned the successful execution of maintenance can serve as a protection for service. Efficiency and accountability in the procurement and utilization of resources is vital for the survival of human service organisations. Without these activities, the very basis of the organisation, and its service is threatened. This relationship in which maintenance supports service, is optimal for the quality of service outcome. However overly emphasized maintenance management can have serious implications for the human service organisation.

Within the management process there is in a sense, a 'natural' conflict between service and maintenance due to the norms that each maintains and the objectives that each pursues. Service particularly human service is not the most efficient endeavour, nor the most tangible or easily objectified. Yet it is objectification and tangibility that are the foundations of maintenance management. As a result some conflict is possible and even probable. How this conflict is manifested in a given organisation depends upon the persons involved and how the maintenance and service tasks are organized and divided. An imbalance toward maintenance can and often does threaten organisational optimization. Consider organizational decision making, for example. We have indicated that congruence should exist if service outcome is to be enhanced and that other considerations such as value elements though present and important, should not predominate as the basis of decision making. If the values present are the values that support the given profession and the optimal application of its technology, there is little basis for conflict. However the pursuit of maintenance objectives may be contradictory to professional values and capability considerations. Such a clash may lead to the appearance of political elements as well. Consider an agency that is under pressure from a major funding source to treat more patients in its outpatient clinic. The agency's current policy is to treat not only the outpatient clinic. The agency's current policy is to treat not only the principal individual patient but to have ongoing collateral contacts with the individual's family. The agency's staff maintains that it is impossible to treat the patient effectively without seeing the family members as well; the funding source maintains that more primary clients could be treated if these secondary contacts were to be reduced.

In this situation, there is a clash between maintenance and service perspectives. The resolution should be decided on the merits of the issue from a service capability perspective but clearly that is not always possible. A balance must be maintained. If this and several issues like it are decided solely on the basis of efficiency, the organisation will begin to co-opt its own service effectiveness. Therefore the managerial structure in a human service organisation must evolve a balance in order to mediate service and maintenance management.

Another example further illustrates the point. Consider the maintenance tasks involved in resource procurement which require a particular kind of reportage and persuasion that may tax the value and capability elements of an organisation and which may result in many dilemmas. Funds may be available, for example, to a given human service organisation, only if it undertakes a new type of service that it is not capable of providing effectively. From a capability perspective, then, acquiring the grant will probably not produce effective service and may even detract from the organisation's current service delivery. Yet the money may be considerable and receiving it promises expansion of the organisation's domain. The decision must be reduced to "Go for the money now and we'll worry about the capability later" as opposed to "let's reject the money because we really cant's deliver the service." Most human service organisations would indeed pursue the grant and many agencies have be built on such pursuit. Co-operation then can be there result of such an imbalance between maintenance and service management. This is further aggravated by the fragmentation between management and service practitioners caused by the dominance of maintenance management. To the extent that management views itself as primarily involved with maintenance and removed from service—in short a generic perspective of management—the overall patterns of service in a given organisation remain unattended and unplanned opening the possibility for the emergence of the kinds of dysfunctional patterns suggested by the frame work of Part I. In such cases, the organisation's effectiveness is diminished its, very reason for being is threatened its contribution to the alleviation of social problems decreased, and its role and the strengthening of the social welfare institution rendered inert. The concept of management viewed solely or to a large extent as maintenance, is not sufficient to lead the human service organisation to optimization and patterns of most effective service. A finely conceived and aggressively pursued service management, balanced carefully with maintenance management, can contribute to the optimization of a human service organisation and help that organisation achieve some degree of effectiveness leading it to outcomes that actually work.

To strengthen the social welfare institution and make the programs and policies more effective in the organisation in which they are implemented the development and application for service management and its integration with maintenance management is a necessity. The next four chapters consider four central functions of human service management; budgeting program evaluation staff development and community relations. Before presenting these four functions it is necessary first to considers a dynamic central to all management—the trade off mechanism.

The strategy of management: The trade-off mechanism

Thus far we have dealt with the necessity, on the part of management to be aware of the structures and processes of a human service organisation Much of the actual execution of management requires interaction with people. It is important before considering the functional areas of management to consider the strategies that human service management must pursue in order to carry out those functions.

In the course of performing the functions of management those in managerial positions will need to pursue strategies and propose certain actions plans and policies. Each managerial 'move' will utilize some combination of organisational components and will require the cooperation of members who are part of these components. On what basis can the manager determine which 'moves' are appropriate in terms of their effect on the organisation and its members and how the organisation will respond? No law or principle governing each possible situation faced by human service management can be given, but a general approach can be derived form the concept of the trade-off mechanism.

Profits, rewards and costs

George C. Homans has provided considerable insight into the actions and interactions of individuals and groups. Homan's work has been characterised as exchange theory. This basis of exchange theory is the following equation:

profit = reward — cost

On the surface this equation appears as a simple explanation of the basic economics of a business; profit equals rewards, or income, minus costs or what the businessmen invest. But Ho-mans extends this prospective to social phenomena, that is, to interactions among individuals and groups, and suggests that such interaction can be analyzed through an application of this formula. Consider by way of illustration the exchange between a small store and its customers. If the store sells a particular item at a certain price, that price minus the cost at which the store initially obtained the item, must produce a reasonable profit for the store. This "trade-off mechanism" between reward and cost and profit must be continuously assessed in order that it be judged "worth it". The customer has his or her own trade-off mechanism. The customer must pay a cost in order to gain a reward and must determine whether the profit is worth it: is the item worth the cost? Homans maintains that relationships among individuals and groups function in much the same manner in that both parties have a notion of their own trade-off mechanisms and the exchange between then is based on an interaction that is profitable to both. Homans argues that "no exchange continues unless both parties are making a profit."

In human interaction the trade-off mechanisms and exchange are more difficult to calculate than in the case of money. What is rewarding and ultimately profitable to one person or group may not be so to others, and the same is true of cost. Rewards for some individuals may lie in the political realm; for others in upholding values or in technological achievement. One organisational members might compromise his order values in order to gain politically; for others the cost with peers and colleagues of such a political gain might prove too high. The pursuit of one's values might also eventually prove too costly and this realization might cause an individual to alter his or her behaviour.

This is not meant to imply that people consciously behave in this calculative manner at all times. Trade-offs may not be apparent and individuals land groups may unconsciously participate in unprofitable exchanges which are not in their self interest. Much political functioning in an organisation, for example, is based on the assumption that the "opponent" does not understand the true cost of a given exchange and when he or she does realize it, it will be too late for him or her to act—the costs will be higher than anticipated. This is the essence of one upmanship Homans believes that given a rational process exchanges can be understood and their course predicted on the basis of understanding the trade-offs involved. It is impossible in Homans' view to understand the dynamics of interrelationships without understanding these trade-off and exchanges.

For example, in a graduate school of social work or any graduate school program, a number of students each year appear for the first day of classes. Each student has gone through some calculation and has arrived at some trade-off regarding his attendance. Obviously, or her the rewards costs and profits are different in each case, but the process is similar and each student anticipates a profitable balance. The reward may be learning, it may be advancement in a job, it any be entering a profession in which one can pursue one's values or a combination of these and other rewards. The cost may involve money, time, family responsibilities, aversion to school, or not doing something else that is positive and rewarding. In all cases, however the profit has been judged to be "worth it." As their exchange with the school unfolds the students assess the rewards, cost, and profits. Some may ultimately decide that the profits are too small and leave perhaps expressing the decision in Homansian terms; "I"m not getting enough out of it. In each case a new trade-off has been perceived which affects the basic exchange. The same dynamic holds for smaller decisions such as which course to take. Each student has a trade off worked out for course selection, in which the possible rewards might range from the instructor's reputation for knowledge, to the fact that he or she assigns only a few page of reading for the semester and no paper. It does seem clear that alterations of such course requirements will change the prospective trade-offs of the students.

Similar calculations of trade-offs can also be applied to other kinds of endeavours. In applying a technology a physician requires an exacting knowledge of trade-offs but most medications or surgical procedures carry some risk of side effects that is costs for the patient. The reward in this case is an improvement in the patient's health. The difference between the rewards and cost must represent a significant profit for the patient in order for the procedure to be undertaken. In some cases the rewards and costs of a given procedure may be extremely close but the cost of not undertaking it may be the determining factor.

The concept of the trade-off is by no means limited to discrete individual interactions but can also apply to patterns of interaction extending over time. The following three propositions from Homans illustrate this point;

> For all actions taken by persons the more often a particular action of a person is rewarded the more likely he is to perform that action.
>
> The more valuable to a person is the result of this action, the more likely he is to perform the action.
>
> The more often in the recent past a person has received a particular reward the less valuable any further unit of that reward becomes for him.

We will return to these propositions later in the chapter in the discussion of their application to managerial strategies.

Trade-off and exchange then can accumulate over time and come to represent an ongoing process, the dynamics of which can be both complex and subtle. Understanding and utilizing these concepts can prove extremely useful in devising the strategies necessary to carry out the functions described in the following chapters.

Trade-offs and the functions of human service management

In a human service organisational context trade-offs and exchanges occur continually between individuals groups and organisations. As those with managerial responsibility perform the functions described in the following chapters they must maintain a thorough understanding of the nature of trade-offs and exchanges that operate between different organisational members and different organisational and interorganisational components. These individuals need to understand the costs rewards and profits of all these elements as they intercalate and as they are viewed not only from the management perspective but also from other viewpoints as well. The manager needs to be able to discern shifts in exchanges and trade-offs in order to trace the response and implications of various managerial policies, programs, and initiatives. In short each significant managerial initiative brings changes to trade-offs and exchanges and without a clear understanding of these, it is nearly impossible to plan and effectively manage in human service Organisations.

Given an understanding of the currents of trade-offs in a human service organisational setting and the knowledge that any managerial initiative will alter these trade-offs, the overall strategy for management is: to govern these currents in such a way as to make the trade-offs and exchanges functional to organisational optimization and the services effectiveness of the organisation.

Trade-offs and exchanges are present in a human service organisation as the staff acts and interacts. The issue is not whether they are present but rather what is the substance of the trade-offs, the content of the profits rewards and costs. The objective of management is to ensure that the content of the trade-offs enhances service effectiveness. This is a subtle process in which mistakes can be costly. If the trade-offs or exchanges of a particular managerial move are assessed incorrectly, the results could be highly dysfunctional in terms of service. Yet to stimulate and maintain meaningful change in the organisation which has a lasting effect on the service product, this process must be executed with a high degree of proficiency.

To further illustrate the concept of the trade-off mechanism, let us briefly consider this mechanism in the context of the elements of throughput described in part I. As noted, various patterns of throughput functioning can bring about organisational cooperation. A significant factor contributing to this co-operation as we have seen is insufficient service resources. In addition cooperation is maintained through patterns of exchange and trade-offs internal to the organisation that lead functioning away from optimization.

In decision making for example capability elements that would contribute most directly to service outcome as the basis of decisions can give way to political elements that are pursued for their own end. One type of service component may be preferable to another in terms of overall organisational capability, but another service may be chosen for the expansion of staff because this component has yielded on some point in the past, and it is now "their turn" to receive a reward. Such trade-offs often detract from optimization but they are common.

Goal displacement itself may also be fuelled by trade-off considerations. Certain operative goals may be maintained because they are to the advantage of individuals or groups in the organisation as in the previous example of the mental hospital where custodial goals have come to displace therapeutic goals. As noted, the hospital as an accountable sub unit of a larger system requires, some form of assessment mechanism and that mechanism may be based on custodial accomplishments. Therefore the director in charge of a particular ward or building may see to it that custodial activities and functions are successfully carried out because the director's rewards and profits in the context of the Organisation's assessment will be derived from contodial results. His or her costs, alternatively will derive from unsuccessful custodial functioning. Thus a series of major patient disturbances may cost the director more than will patients failure to get well. Hence the strict pursuit of operative goals is the most profitable course, because the Organisation is conducted that way. This is not to imply that this particular director is necessarily an extremely insensitive person but rather that in the normal course of events most people will pursue the course most profitable to them.

The same formula holds true for the exercise of authority. If a superior perceives that his or her most profitable course lies in exercising authority based on position rather than ability that person may do so. A supervisor may find that allowing his or her subordinates to contribute as equals is too threatening and too costly people in authority positions often conclude that the rewards of initiating collegial relationships do not outweigh the cost of relinquishing some of their authority in the process. From a service perspective it is in fields with minimally developed technologies that a collegial perspective is probably most desirable since clear-cut gradations in professional ability are difficult to discern. Yet, it is in just this situation that the superior is less likely to give up authority and initiate a collegial relationship because he or she may feel most threatened by his or her lack of sound professional ability. This is a great dilemma in human service organisations and very costly in terms of service because the potential for a ritualized authority based on position is great. Innovative or alternative technological approaches may be suppressed or go unrewarded because of an inflexible structure. "Standing on rank" may become very common and technological activities may be rigidly controlled by superiors.

In these and other throughput processes, management must guide the reward system of the organisation in order to influence behaviour in the direction of optimization and effective service. Here maintenance management and service management can be closely integrated. Maintenance resources constitute a major source of reward that can be drawn upon by management. It is important that the internal dispersal of these resources be based on capability and not merely political trade-offs. To the extent possible, advancement in the organisation, not only in terms of position but also recognition of various kinds, must be based on contribution of the organisation, official goals and its service outcome rather than on the ability of members to successfully engage in purely political operations. The costs of not contributing technologically must be high and the rewards for doing so must also be high, so that the organisational dynamics will move toward optimization. In short, advancement of individuals in the organisation must be closely tied to their technological achievement. Obviously ongoing activities that are designed to achieve this vary with many organisational factors one of the most important being size. In larger organisations, more formal means, such as policy and program initiative, will have the most impact whereas in smaller organisations the process is characterized to a greater degree interpersonal contact.

Consider the three elaborations of the exchange theory previously mentioned: the success the value and the deprivation satiation proportions. The success proposition which suggests that a person is more likely to perform an act the more he or she's rewarded for it, illustrates a number of points. The rewards need to be based on the person's contribution to service effectiveness. But in order to maximize this dynamic a system of rewards is necessary and not merely an undisciplined occasional reward. Organisational mechanisms should be designed which continually reward members for positive contributions. This might be a part of staff evaluations, a variety of ad hoc and on going tasks that are important to the organisation, or the satisfaction that is gained when a person's participation and input become part of organisational policy. Although this may appear evident, is an infrequent practice, particularly on a systematic basis in most human service organisations. The task of devising strategies that include ongoing rewards based on service effectiveness is difficult but vital, and must be put of a management perspective. The trade offs as perceived by organisational members need to be 'tilted' in favour of contributing to service effectiveness in order to ensure that members gain rewards from positive contribution and not form dysfunctional organisational behaviour.

The value proposition stating that the more valuable an action to a person, the more likely he or she is to perform it, is also relevant and is related to the success proposition. What constitutes value for the members of a human service organisation is an important question for it is as we have noted the basis of an individual's trade-off mechanism. The manager of a human service organisation must set the value tone so that the pursuit of service effectiveness will be perceived as valuable or rewarding at all levels of an organisation. This of course, is not totally attainable but it must be continually sought. A human service profession should socialize the practitioner to service and to the importance of effective, quality care. However, as has been indicated previously, when a practitioner functions in the context of an organisation it is possible for socialization to work in a negative direction Where that individual once valued service he or she may now come to place greater value on behaviour ranging from ventilating hostility against the organisation to learning the ropes in order to get ahead. Management must attempt to minimize such behaviour by utilizing the reward system to enhance the influence of professional values and norms dedicated to service effectiveness.

The deprivation-satiation proposition illustrates how difficult these tasks are to accomplish. This proposition posits that the more often a person receives a given reward the less valuable it is to him or her. The repetition of the same unit of a given reward even if it is accomplishing the purpose of increasing the service effectiveness of the organisation, will not yield a consistent result over time. Different kinds of rewards will be needed in order to perpetuate an appropriately oriented reward system. Therefore in human service management, the strategy must continually be altered in order to ensure maximal result. It is this need to alter strategy that makes human service management so demanding an endeavour.

What has been presented is an overview of the use of trade off mechanisms in the enhancement of service effectiveness. The ongoing assessment of trade-offs and the ability to utilize the appropriate initiative to elicit the desired response in terms of service effectiveness is a skill which is often perceived and developed by those who are successful in management as an intuitive derive process. The skill is utilized not only in planning but also in both formal and informal interaction. The need to function in this calculative manner is an important aspect of management. Whereas the inability to function politically may not be essential to the clinician in performing treatment tasks, it is necessity to those who perform management functions in a human service setting. Being able to analyze the human service organisation or to understand the functioning of management, as presented in this chapter is not sufficient. Operationalization of the analysis and execution of the functions and strategies are required, and this necessitates strategic functioning such as timing what to trade, how far to go whom to utilize and so forth .

It is vital that an important point not be overlooked. These activities must be considered as a means to improving services and should not become ends in themselves. The tendency to do so can be a serious problem in management. The strategies presented in this chapter should be pursued only as they contribute to the functions and not for the self-interest of the manager or others in the organisation. In clinical role the clinician must serve the client's needs and not his or her own. This is true of the manager as well. The client's needs and the organisational activities that affect those needs must be the goal which is served. In addition, the means must be integrated with that goal. This constitutes the ethics of human service management.

Managerial styles: Instrumental and expressive

We have considered the functions of human service management and the basis on which management must plan strategies in order to carry out these functions. The final subject area in this chapter concerns the style of the manager and the patterns of behaviour that he or she exhibits in executing these functions and carrying out the strategies. There are two general kinds of style models, both of which are important in carrying out the objectives of management presented in this book. The first is the expressive and the second is the instrumental. The expressive style emphasizes affect, human relationships, and interaction; the treatment of organisational members as fellow humans rather than as instruments designed to execute particular tasks. The instrumental style focuses on task accomplishment. The emphasis is on what the organisational member can do in the pursuit of the organisation's formal activity. Both of these styles are important and necessary in the functioning of human service organisations. Who in management plays each, at which time, and to what extent depends on organisational position personality and on other factors. One common pattern is an inside person and an outside person. An outside person is often the head of the Organisation who generally performs the expressive role. A political candidate is a good example of this. This handshaking the smile the backslapping and the attempt at being well liked are all part of an expressive-oriented style. Yet the candidate must have an 'inside person' a 'nuts and bolts' person, who tends to the 'hard' aspects of the campaign. This person need not have an effusive personality because he or she deals with administrative matters and the style is instrumental. Obviously one person can assume both roles but the conventional approach is that at least in public the number two person is more instrumental and the head person is more expressive.

The distinction between expressive and instrumental management styles has grown with the development of management theories. At the turn of the century, Frederick Taylor founded what he called "scientific management." This was a highly in instrumental concept that viewed organisational members as cogs in a machine designed to be as efficient as possible. Time and Motion Studies originated from this approach and were designed to answer the question, What physical movements on the part of the workers are most efficient in production? Scientific management dealt with such ideas as the optimal span of control of a manager and the proper distribution of task. The whole notion was geared toward manufacturing plants of the era. The Human Relations School developed in response to this approach beginning with the Hawthorne study, conducted during 1929-32 at a Western General Electric plant to investigate the process of work. The basic finding of this study was that other factors, informal in nature can contribute much to productivity and to efficiency. Group norms, personality factors, loyalty and so forth affect workers as much or more than some of the structured measures and considerations of the scientific management school Today much of management theory in essence has become a blend of the two with a stress on both structural approaches and the more intangible but equally important, expressive aspects as part of job satisfaction and productivity.

The human service organisation and its resources

In order to begin to assess systematically the functioning of human service organisations consideration must be given to the kinds of raw materials. resources, or inputs that are required. All formal complex organisations untilize what can be called maintenance resources which include founding equipment supplies, a physical plant, and so forth. These resources are necessary, to ensure the survival of an organisation. A human service organisation however because of the uniqueness of its organisational product requires a second kind of resource. This can be termed a service resource which is derived from the existence and availability of a specific type of expertise designed to alleviate the given social problem with which the organisation deals. It is this kind of resource that forms the basis and ultimately determines the effectiveness of an organisation, service product. Without sufficient service resources an organisation cannot deliver an effective service product, despite the presence of an adequate quantity of maintenance resources

The procurement and efficient disposal of maintenance resources is the basic of maintenance management. The procurement and overall effective application of the service resources constitutes service management. The management of maintenance resources is a subject that has been extensively explored, particularly in the areas of business and public administration. An integrated and developed concept of the management of service resources on the other hand has received little attention. Hence the emphasis through out this work is on service resources and their management. Maintenance resources are considered in the context of their effect on service outcome. The ultimate purpose of human service management is to promote and enhance effective service, therefore efficiency and maintenance must be viewed as a means to that end, rather than as goals in themselves.

The service resource

The state of a human service technology

A useful concept that helps to clarify the notion of a service resource is a human service technology, which may be defined as the sum total of the knowledge, procedures, and techniques that, when applied in a given human service field, will yield consistent, desired, and predictable results. Charles Perrow an organisational analyst, has developed several criteria for what may be considered a model of a highly developed human service technology:

1. Some knowledge of a nonrandom cause-and

effect relationship is, required, that is, the techniques lead to the performance of acts which, for known or unknown reasons, cause a change under specific conditions.

2. There is some system of feedback such that the consequences of the acts can be assessed in an objective manner.
3. It is possible to secure repeated demonstrations of the efficacy of the acts.
4. There is an acceptable reasonable, and determinant range of tolerance that is the proportion of the successes must be estimated and even though the proportion might be small, it is judged high enough to continue the activity.
5. The techniques can be communicated sufficiently so that most persons with appropriate preliminary training can be expected to master the techniques and perform them under acceptable limits of tolerance.

Taken together these criteria represent an ideal technology in the highest state of development. Such criteria are useful as standards for assessing the state of a given technology at a given time. Technologies may approach all of these criteria in which case they are highly developed, they may manifest few or none in which case they are minimally developed or they may reflect varying degrees of development. To understand the concept of human service technology it is therefore important that it be viewed as a continuous variable or factor The important consideration is not whether a technology is present but to what degree it is present making it a continuous variable. It is a rare human service in which no technology whatever is present and an equally rare situation in which a human technology is fully developed. This continuous concept can be visualized as follows with most if not all actual human service technologies falling between the two poles.

Every organisation employs some kind of technology in order to execute the functions it is designed to carry out. In a manufacturing plant technology is typically tangible in that the process of assembling the elements results in a concrete product, be it clothing automobiles or toothpaste. This kind of technology is generally characterised by a high degree of routinization once the operational system is in place the tasks become clear the causative relationships apparent, the process highly repetitive and the product standardized. Some technologies are so perfected that human input becomes marginal. The spaceflights are a good example. Rather than being commanded as in much science fiction, by a human being who acted often by instinct and in crises, quickly developed and applied a new theoretical break through the spaceflights were dominated by a computerized technology that left little to chance. So routinised became the technology that the excitement for television audiences, become increasingly diminished as the number of flights increased.

The technology of human service is quite different. What actually occurs between a patient and a therapist in a mental health setting, or a social worker and a client in a drug abuse program a worker and a trainee in a manpower training program or a caseworker and a public assistance recipient in a social services program constitutes a technology characterized by elements that are difficult to control. Unlike the highly routinized technology of manufacturing, which deals with inanimate objects, human service technology concerns changes in human beings and is therefore far less tangible and definable. Nevertheless the product of a human service organisation is its service effectiveness and technology represents the vital component that constitutes the necessary raw material ultimately leading to the formulation of that product.

Although there has been some research linking technology to other aspects of organisational functioning, there has, unfortunately, been little work attempting to analyze and compare different human service technologies. Great differences in technological development are apparent. Health-related technology, particularly surgery, is relatively more developed in its techniques and specialized procedures than is community organisation, for example, which has only progressed to the point of descriptive categories of professional functioning and the development of role models for practice.

The degree of development of a given human service technology used by a given human service

Organisation is a crucial factor in the eventual quality of its service. If little is known about a particular human service problem and how to treat or alleviate it, then it will be difficult for a human service organisation for function in a consistent effective manner no matter how efficient it may be how much rhetoric surrounds it initiation or how much public support it may command. What is achieved can most probably be attributed to serendipitous and inconsistent techniques.

The first factor, then, in understanding how the ultimate quality of the service product of a human service organisation is determined lies in the state of development of the technology that the organisation employs. In order to understand the service resources available to the organisation the manager must understand the capabilities and limitations of the given technology. The manager must consider for example the following kinds of questions concerning the technology.

1. Is the technology exacting and routinized?
2. Is it abstract and intangible ?
3. Are advances and modifications in the technology frequent?
4. Is there concrete evidence of its efficacy and effectiveness?
5. Are its elements easy or difficult to measure?
6. Are its elements easily communicated?

None of these nor similar kinds of questions that

serve to help clarify the nature of a given human service technology have ready answers. But without an approach and consideration to these kinds of questions it is difficult to perceive how a human service manager might proceed in enhancing the service product of an organisation.

The degree to which human service technology is possessed by practitioners

The state of development of a human service technology does not in itself. Constitute a service resource. There may, in fact exist a technology at a sufficiently high state of development to provide some degree of effective service but if a sufficient number of practitioners who are trained to untilize it are unavailable to a given organisation the technology itself is of little use in actual service delivery. Therefore, the possession of the technology by practitioners who are available to the organisation becomes an important factor. The focal points for technological development and training are the human service professions and their educational institutions. In graduate schools of social work, for example the technology of social casework which is practiced in a great variety of human service settings is taught to future professionals. To what degree is the state of the technology actually transmitted to these students? Clearly, factors are present in an educational process that can cause the nature of what transpires to be less than adequate thereby adversely affecting a future parctitioners preparation and ultimately reducing his other technological possession This issue is primarily an educational one but it has a significant effect on the level of practice that takes place in human service organisations. If the educational institution can transmit most of the technological elements or a framework through which these elements can be assembled by future practitioners then the eventual quality of service in the organisation in which these practitioners eventually practice is maximized. Of course the acquisition of technology by no means ends in school and much is acquired 'on the job' but the educational process can provide the basis of professional identity and socialization that depends largely upon the acquisition of technological knowledge and skill.

As in the case of the state of technology it is unlikely that a practitioner of human services will possess no degree of technology, nor is it likely that he or she would possess such knowledge to the point at which there is no opportunity for further development. Therefore the degree of possession is clearly another continuous variable.

Thus the second factor involved in understanding how effective service is derived is the degree of technology possessed by the practitioners who provide the service. A human service manager needs to consider the following kinds of questions:

1. Is a profession involved in the technology? Do the formal educational credentials relate to a significant degree to the actual carrying out of tasks. Does the profession have different gradation levels and do these levels relate significantly to the possession of ability?

2. Does the knowledge on which the technology is based include different formalized schools of thought and are there controversies in the field? Are such schools and controversies manifested by the practitioners of the Organisation?

3. Can the degree to which the technology is possessed be determined and evaluated? Are standards of assessment part of the profession? Is an assessment on the level of training and the nature of the professional background available?

It is both the state of a human service technology and its possession by practitioners, then that provide the basis for understanding the service resources of a human service organisation. In understanding how an organisation derives its product, therefore, the human service manager needs to understand these two factor in the context of a given organisation. A knowledge and assessment of these "raw materials" that compose the service resources of the organisation is a necessary step in understanding the totality of how the service product is produced.

The availability of service resources thus constitutes the input in the process culminating in a service product.

11 Health Care of Laboratory Personnel

Laboratory personnel particularly those working in departments of microbiology may be exposed to the risk of infection in the course of their daily work. That infection do occur from time to time is well documented. Sometimes it is the individual worker who becomes ill and in this case, if the infecting agent is common in the community, proof that the infection occurred in the laboratory may be difficult to obtain. Occasionally many staff may be infected at the same time and if the organism is known to be absent from the community then the source, the laboratory, is apparent. Such an incident indeed took place in Michigan, USA in 1938/39 when 45 clinical cases of brucellosis occurred in association with a laboratory. The infecting organism *Brucella melitensis* had not been isolated in that territory in recent years and all milk consumed by those infected was known to have been pasteurized. Rarely, infection of a laboratory employee leads to spread of disease in the community, as happened with smallpox in London in 1973. Such clear-cut examples of hazards in the laboratory do not fortunately, occur very often but now that infectious diseases have decreased in importance in the western world such outbreaks can have profound repercussions. There is foremost the personal tragedy of deaths such as occurred in the London smallpox outbreak, or there may be chronic ill-health which follows infection with brucellosis. In addition there is inevitably an over-reaction in the community which may result in the imposition of stricter regulations over a wide field of laboratory work. In some instances such regulations may lead to safer working conditions and should be accepted and implemented by those concerned. In other instances regulations across the board can lead to restrictions of activities in fields where hazards are more imaginary than real and thus curtail research and routine work to the detriment of patient care. At the lowest level such restrictions are seen by workers to be unnecessary and are therefore ignored, bringing all safety regulations into disrepute. For all these reasons it is essential that management and worker should co-operate to reduce hazards in the laboratory. One aspect of the reduction of hazard is to look after the health of the laboratory worker. It is the objective of this chapter to outline the steps which should be taken in this direction. In the UK an Act of Parliament The Health and Safety at Work etc. Act 1974 has clearly defined responsibilities in this field. A Health and Safety Commission is responsible for policy decisions which are translated into action by inspectors of the Health and Safety Executive.

Such inspectors have the power to visit and advise on safety in all occupations including laboratories. In this they have support in law. In addition and probably more important than the legal aspects of health and safety at work, management usually in the form of the director of the laboratory, has a moral responsibility to look after the health of his staff. On the other hand each individual worker has a legal and moral responsibility for safety, for his actions may imperil his fellow workers or members of the community in which he lives.

Further to the Health and Safety at Work Act of 1974 new regulations in this field came into force in the UK in 1989. These are the Control of Substances Hazardous to Health Regulations requiring an employer not to expose employees to any substance hazardous to health unless an assessment has been made of the risks and steps taken to mitigate against these. Employees must be informed of the risks and the precaution that must be taken. Clearly, these Regulations include chemicals and micro-organisms, methods of handling, and in particular ventilation systems and biological safety cabinets.

As in all respects of Health and Safety, the keeping of records is of primary importance.

The employer although responsible, is able to delegate implementation of these Regulations to the Laboratory Director who will be assisted by the Laboratory Safety Officer and the Laboratory Safety Committee.

As these Regulations apply to the whole hospital as well as to laboratories the Health Authorities may appoint a Coordinator and Control of Hazardous Substances Team..

Fitness for employment

The health care of laboratory personnel should commence when the candidate first presents himself or herself for a job. No interview is complete without.

(a) the candidate's medical questionnaire;

(b) An explanation of the work and possible hazards involved.

The medical questionnaire

Some authorities require a full medical examination report before appointment. There are occasionally indications for this to be done but such routine examinations are not always a necessity for civilian appointment. It is often just as rewarding to ask the candidate to answer a series of questions on his health and to indicate that untrue statements may lead to the loss of the job. It is rare for the candidate to lie. The important questions include age, height and weight, and these should be compared with tables showing the normal distribution. A marked difference, over 10% from the normal, should lead to examination by a medically qualified practitioner. It is essential to establish previous medical history with particular emphasis on mental outlook, a history of allergies or skin diseases and previous accidents or operations. The introspective individual may allow imaginary hazards to prey upon his mind, the allergic may not be able to work with animals and the individual who has had a severe accident may be physically incapable of certain duties. Drugs should be declared. The candidate on immunosuppressive drugs in unsuitable for work in a laboratory. The vaccination history is important. Those who have never received any form of immunization may be in this situation becausc of the attitude adopted by their parents, but it does not means that they are themselves opposed to such policies. The question should be asked either on the form or at interview.

A radiograph of the chest may be indicated but certainly a question should be asked about a vaccination against tuberculosis. If the individual has had BCG it is as well to examine the site to establish without doubt that this has been done.

Variations from the normal should be investigated sympathetically. Some 8% of men are red/blue colour blind but for women the incidence is less than 1%. This should not necessarily exclude a good candidate for employment in a laboratory. The intelligent individual soon learns to compensator for this minor defect and many good technical workers recognize the tubercle bacillus through a microscope as much by its shape and size as by its colour. Even epilepsy has not debarred all laboratory workers in the past. Providing the condition is well controlled, or the individual has rare attacks with adequate premonitory, signs he or she can perform laboratory duties successfully.

An explanation of the work and possible hazards involved

This is an important element of the interview. The candidate's reaction to the need to receive a series of vaccinations should be judged. The requirement for the worker to be vaccinated should be clearly stated and the candidate should not be appointed if objections or doubts are raised. The attitude adopted to the prospect of being involved in experimental work with animals should also be explored. Both these questions can save a considerable amount of trouble at a later date.

On employment

The employee's medical questionnaire should be filed and a medical record card completed bearing important details from the questionnaire. This card should be designed to display the complete immunization history. For the small laboratory this procedure is adequate, but it requires a conscientious and dedicated approach to health care for these cards must all be checked at intervals year after year to ensure that the employee is offered booster vaccine doses at the proper intervals. A much more efficient method applicable to larger laboratories is to place the individual's medical history on a computer with safeguards to ensure that only those authorized can recall the information. Using modern data-handling equipment it is possible to have available each month a list of those individuals who require booster doses of vaccine during that calendar month. This leads to greater efficiency in recall and it also spreads the load for the doctor who is called upon to give a few injections each month throughout the year instead of dealing with larger numbers at infrequent intervals. This has the added advantage of making the employee feel that this being treated as an individual instead of one of a herd. The shrewd doctor will take advantage of this situation as it gives him time to make inquiries concerning health and personal problems and thus to anticipate and often deal with difficulties before they assume major proportions.

The medical record card should display the employee's name and address, his or her next of kin and the name of his medical practitioner. When this is completed, and before any arrangements are made for immunization, a letter should go to the medical practitioner telling him that the individual has started work in a microbiological laboratory. This will be filed with the patient's records and should alert the doctor if his patient develops an unexplained fever. The letter should also explain that the employee will shortly be offered immunization against a variety of infectious diseases unless the doctor writes to register any objection or would prefer to administer the prophylaxis himself. It is rare for any such objection to be raised if this procedure is followed, but problems can arise if the employee is immunized without prior notice to the doctor.

Two further steps should be issued with a personal card to be taken at the stage. The employee should be carried at all times. This card should show the name and address of the holder and the name and telephone number of his doctor. In addition, the card should state where he or she works and the telephone number of one or more senior members of the medical staff of the laboratory. This card should be produced to the attending physician if the laboratory scientist is taken ill. Such a card will alert the physician to the possibility of a laboratory infection and enable him to discuss the case with laboratory staff who will know if indeed any such hazards exist.

The second step is the collection of a specimen of blood to provide serum for a double purpose. The serum can be screened for the presence of antibody to a variety of infection diseases and will be discussed under these headings. The specimen can then be stored for retrieval at a later date, to provide a 'baseline' specimen if the employee falls ill.

Finally the new recruit should where possible be given an *induction course.*

The amount of time which can be allocated to an *induction course* for newly appointed personnel will vary with the size of the laboratory. The small diagnostic laboratory taking one or two new workers at any one time may be unable to allocate any formal teaching at this stage. It is useful to attach the new staff to the laboratory safety officer for a brief period so the importance of observing safety precautions is instilled from the first day. Safety is largely an attitude of mind and the new recruit should be clearly shown that such precautions are taken seriously in the laboratory. In larger laboratories one or more days may be set aside for an induction course and this although emphasizing safety, may be used with advantage to allow the recruit to find his way about in what may be a complex and unfamiliar world. Such a course should include lectures or demonstrations on:

(a) laboratory hazards with an introduction to the literature on the subject;

(b) legal aspects of safety at work;

(c) the use of protective equipment such as safety cabinets and clothing, e.g. respirators and Martindale suits;

(d) how to write a protocol for a work programme so that potential hazards can be highlighted and obviated;

(e) how to handle animals safely;

(f) specialist fields such as chemicals and gases, if these are relevant;

(g) the safe transit of specimens as laid down by the Health Services Advisory Committee.

Finally, consideration should be given to offering protective vaccination against the following diseases.

Tuberculosis

Laboratory-acquired tuberculosis was first shown to be a problem in the UK by Reid, who demonstrated in the early 1950s that laboratory workers were from 2 to 5 times more likely to contract tuberculosis than a control group. It had been known for many years that this disease was a hazard to those who handled clinical material but this work was the first to use a control group. Similar figures were shown in France and Canada and again in the UK 20 years later. In retrospect it is disturbing that such a hazard should have persisted into the 1970s for the dangers to young nurses of contact with cases of open tuberculosis had been recognized for a generation. The role of BCG vaccination in prevention has also been well documented. The incidence of tuberculosis in the general population, although falling steadily over the years, remains appreciable. In England and Wales in 1987, 4000 cases occurred in population of approximately 50 million. Such cases are well investigated, it being usual to send at least three specimens of sputum to the microbiological laboratory for culture for M.tuberculosis and subsequently to send specimens at monthly intervals to determine the effect of treatment and to confirm that the organism remains sensitive to antituberculous drugs. The development of antibiotic resistance may also require may also require further laboratory investigations, Routine procedures of this type ensure a steady flow of potentially infectious material into the laboratory. The following precautions should be taken;

(a) Technical procedures should be used which are known to be least hazardous. Work should be done in safety cabinets in a room designated for this purpose. Facilities such as disposable caps, gowns and handwashing facilities should be available.

(b) Staff should be tuberculin tested and their BCG status should be known. It is not sufficient to ask if vaccination has been done the vaccination site should be inspected. If evidence of successful vaccination is present this should be recorded together with the results of the tuberculin test. There is good evidence that the administration of BCG gives long-lasting immunity to those living in the UK even if their skin sensitivity has waned. If no typical scar is present it should be assumed that no vaccination has been done and BCG should be given. Unvaccinated staff with little induration with the Mantoux test or Heaf test grade II or less should also be vaccinated. Skin reactions greater than those described raise the question of active tuberculosis and further investigation including a chest radiographs will be necessary. It is possible that routine BCG vaccination of school children will soon be stopped in the UK Special groups may continue to be vaccinated and it is reasonable to argue that scientists working with Mycobacteria should be one of these.

Routine chest radiographs are of doubtful value, but the recommendation that they should be done is found in all the codes of practice for the care of the health of laboratory staff. Thus laboratory workers should be encouraged to have repeat chest radiographs at 2-3 year intervals, especially if they work with the agent.

Newly joined staff who have spent their early life overseas should be assessed carefully. BCG has not proved as effective in India as in the West. It is not known if this finding is due to BCG used or to the individual's exposure to related mycobacteria period to vaccination. Until this finding is explained consideration should be given to revaccination even in the presence of evidence of a successful 'take' if this has been given in the tropics.

Enteric disease

Although vaccines have long been available against typhoid fever and paratyphoid A and B only the monovalent typhoid vaccine is now used in UK. This vaccine contains 1000 million salmonella typhi per ml, a much lower dose of organisms than in the polyvalent preparation which used to cause appreciable side-effects. The monovalent vaccine is less troublesome, but whether this is due to the reduction in the numbers of organisms injected or to the absence of the paratyphoid element is not clear. Side-effects do still occur and are more likely the more frequently the vaccine is injected and the older the recipient is. At one time those who had received many booster doses of this vaccine were advised against further injections when they had reached the age of 35. Of course such a recommendation would not apply if exposure to infection was likely.

Typhoid disease has always merited a prominent place in the list of laboratory infections and the danger has been highlighted in recent years in the USA. In America Salmonella typhi is used as a quality control organism and distribution to laboratories there resulted in a number of laboratory infections. In the UK this organism has not been distributed in this way although there is no reason why it should not be so used. Cases of typhoid in the UK, however, rarely exceed 150 each year but even so one death in a laboratory worker was recorded in the 1970s. The vaccine confers some 70-90% protection for a period not exceeding 3 years and booster doses are recommended at that interval after a basic course of two injections at 1-month interval. Medical opinion implies that all laboratory workers should be protected and certainly all those who handle specimens, especially faeces, urine and blood should be inoculated. The administration of the vaccine to all other members of staff including office workers and clearners, can be a difficult decision in countries where the disease is rare. The infection is not airborne and in theory only those handling specimens and cultures should be at risk, but at least five cases have occurred in the USA in laboratory workers who were described as 'merely present in the laboratory'. Vaccination should only be offered after due consideration of the potential hazard.

Live oral typhoid vaccines using the Ty 21a S. typhi strain are not showing as much promise as was hoped and it may be that a genetically engineered vaccine will be used in the future.

Tetanus

A few cases of tetanus infection have occurred in laboratory workers, but this is not a disease which normally presents a hazard in the diagnostic laboratory. In the research laboratory were the toxin may be produced and manipulated the situation may be different. Nevertheless, on general medical grounds no opportunity to vaccinate against tetanus should be missed. The disease, now rare in the West, is still capable of causing death, and in the UK occurs in the young athlete and the middle aged and elderly gardener. The laboratory workers may at sometime or other fall into one of these groups and should; therefore be offered vaccination. Many Europeán countries recommend tetanus vaccination and in some it is compulsory.

The basic course consists of three injections of absorbed tetanus toxoid with an interval of 6-8 weeks between the first and second doses and 6 months between the second and third. Booster does should be given at 5 and 10 years. Many children receive their basic course at an early age combined with diptheria and sometimes with whooping cough. In these instances the laboratory worker will only require a booster dose. Too many booster doses may cause local or even general reactions.

Rubella

All women of child bearing age should be vaccinated against rubella and most countries in Western Europe have a vaccination policy recommending this at ages 12-15 years. The baseline serum collected from newly appointed laboratory workers should, therefore, be examined of evidence of immunity and if such evidence is lacking the live attenuated rubella vaccine should be offered. No reliance should be placed on a history of a rubella like illness in the past as other virus infections are known to cause similar illnesses. The vaccine is contraindicated during the first 3 months of pregnancy and conception should be avoided for 3 months following vaccination. Immunity should be checked 8 weeks after vaccination.

The introduction of measles, mumps rubella vaccine for all children in the UK from 1988 should eventually reduce the risk of rubella infection in pregnant women.

Hepatitis

Hepatitis has been known to occur in laboratory workers for about a century, but it is possible that some of these early cases may have been due to any one of the several different viruses now known to cause this disease. There is, nevertheless, clear evidence of cases occurring following contact with blood and serum, and these were most certainly due to hepatitis B. Blood is not easy to aerosolize and in any case we have no evidence that hepatitis can be spread by the airborne route. It is; however, very easy to splash blood as a result of many manipulations commonly done in the laboratory. Opening containers, especially those with a plug type closure rather than a screw-capped container, is a case in point. Such splashes will contaminate equipment and bench surfaces and thus the clothing and skin. The virus seems able to penetrate into the blood steam via minute cuts sand abrasions, but more dangerous are cuts from sharp instruments such as scalpels and penetrating wounds form needles, from the so-called needle-stick injury. Such minor accidents are not infrequent in laboratories. The virus of hepatitis B is thought to be carried by persistent human carriers forming a vast global reservoir estimated as exceeding 150 million persons. The geographical variation in incidence is wide, ranging from 1 in 800 blood donors in the UK to some 10% of the population in certain parts of Asia and Africa. It follows from this that all blood handled in a laboratory is potentially dangerous and should be treated with a degree of care. Gloves should be worn and protection taken against splashes to the eyes. This may be done by wearing goggles but many prefer to use a safety cabinet which has the added advantage of allowing work to be done behind a glass screen. Needle should be replaced by cannulas, and glass pipettes by plastic disposables. Cuts and scratches should be encouraged to bleed, treated with a disinfectant and covered with a dressing. Technical procedures should be carefully reviewed at intervals to ensure that personnel are handling material with care. Guidelines should be written out and displayed so that no worker has any doubt concerning his responsibility.

In addition to the general guidance already

given the laboratory director should make certain that testing of specimens for hepatitis markers is only done by experienced staff. If the skin is punctured or contamination of mucous membranes is known to have taken place hepatitis B immunoglobulin may be administered. This should only be given if the specimen is known to be positive and the individual is tested to see if he is susceptible. Such a step will not be necessary if all those involved in the testing of such specimens are offered inactivated hepatitis B virus vaccine which has been available since 1982. This vaccine is an inactivated, alum-adsorbed suspension of surface antigen particles. These are purified from human plasma by a combination of physical and chemical procedures followed by a triple process of inactivation each of which are known to inactivate HB and other viruses. The vaccine has now been administered to many persons in various parts of the world and although its safety has been questioned there is no real evidence to raise any doubts. Such questions on the safety of the vaccine arise from the well known fact that the vaccine is derived from human plasma and that some of the donors may have been homosexuals and that cases of AIDS are known to have occurred in the cities where blood was collected to make the vaccine.

In spite of the fact that AIDS may take years to develop there is no evidence to implicate the vaccine in its spread.

The vaccine course consists of three intramuscular doses, the second dose being given after 1 month and the third 6 months after the first. Such course produces antibody in over 90% of those vaccinated and persists for some years; the exact period is yet to be determined.

Since 1986 new genetically engineered vaccine has become available produced by Saccharomyces cerevisiae into which a plasmid has been inserted containing Hepatitis B surface antigen gene. The immune response to the recombinant HB vaccine is satisfactory when given as a three-dose course.

A small proportion of vaccines, less than 10% give a poor response so that when attempting to protect the individual laboratory worker, tests for antibody response may be indicated.

Although the hazards of handling blood are stressed it should be noted that neither in the USA nor in the UK are laboratory workers considered to be a high risk population. Immigrants and refugees from areas of high endemicity those who work with the mentally retarded, homosexuals and drug abusers are all more likely to become infected than those who work in laboratories. In fact, the application of good basic microbiological techniques appears to have caused a fall in the incidence of this disease in those who work in laboratories in the UK. Nevertheless health service staff who develop infection with hepatitis B often fail to identify an accident or incident and the annual incidence of INFECTION in laboratory scientific staff who develop infection with hepatitis B often fail to identify an accident or incident and the annual incidence of infection in laboratory scientific staff was quoted as 37 per 100 000 compared with four among nurses in 1980-84. The comparable figures for 1985-88 are 10 and 2. Clearly there is case for extreme care in handling blood and vaccination should be offered, but in spite of the fact that 5% of the 6,696 cases of hepatitis B in England Wales and Northern Ireland in the years 1980-84 occurred in health care workers, the uptake of vaccination remains poor.

Poliomyelitis

Vaccination against poliomyelitis is recommended in most countries in Western Europe and is compulsory in some. Laboratory workers should be offered and encouraged to be vaccinated, especially if working with faeces as in a routine bacteriology and virology department. Some specialist laboratories handle faeces from abroad including the tropics, and here vaccination is most important.

The vaccine is available as an oral attenuated strain of each of the three types of poliovirus and produces by multiplication a local gut immunity and a serum antibody response. The basic course is three doses at intervals of 6-8 weeks and 4-6 month between the second and third respectively. Contraindications include pregnancy, gastro-intestinal upset and hypersensitivity to antibiotics used in the preparation of the vaccine. A killed vaccine is also available if the live vaccine is contraindicated..

Live vaccine should only be given to laboratory workers if their families are to be vaccinated at the same time as there is a remote chance of enhanced virulence if the vaccine strain is passaged through young siblings. In this situation it is often wiser to use the killed vaccine.

Reinforcing doses are only required if there is no clear history of such a doses being given on leaving school.

Diphtheria

Diphtheria is a rare disease in Western Europe due to the immunization schemes which exist either as recommendations or in compulsory form in different countries. Most children have some basic immunity due to childhood vaccination but few receive booster doses in later life.

Only staff to be exposed to a case of diphtheria or swabs and cultures need to be vaccinated. This can be done using diptheria vaccine depending upon the results of a Schick test. Such a procedure is cumbersome and takes time, and for this reason it will probably be replaced by the use of diphtheria vaccine for adults which is now available. The preparation may be used for the immunization of persons aged over 10 years. Primarily designed for boosting immunity in adults such as laboratory staff it may be given without Schick testing. Neither the immune nor the hypersensitive are likely to experience reactions other than wild side-effects.

Other vaccinations

These should be confined to confined who work with agents in highly specialized laboratories.

Vaccines are against rabies anthrax and botulism as examples.

Rabies immunization is usually done using a three-dose regimen on days 0,7 and 25 of human diploid cell rabies vaccine produced by the Merieux Institute. The usual dose is 0.1 ml by interamuscular injections and this gives adequate titres of antibody. Because of the cost of this vaccine the practice of giving three doses of 0.1 ml by intradermal injection has become common-place but the efficacy of this procedure has been questioned. Doubts arose because of a case of human rabies in a Peace Corps Volunteer working in Kenya and subsequent investigation revealed that the intradermal route did not always result in good protection. If the intradermal route is chosen serological testing should be done 2-3 weeks after immunization and if a titre of less than 1 in 16 recorded, additional doses given until that titre is reached or exceeded.

Anthrax injections in laboratory workers have been reported at intervals since 1914, and Pike has recorded 45 deaths from this disease. The hazard lies in inhalation and is, therefore, largely confined to research institutions where aerosols may be created, particularly by those who have an interest in biological warfare. A vaccine is available prepared from a growth of the sterne strain of anthrax and rendered sterile by filtration and the use of thiomersal as a preservative. The alum-precipitated anthrax antigen is given as a course of four interamuscular injections each of 0.5 ml. The first three doses are given at intervals of 3 weeks and the last dose 6 months later Reinforcing doses are given annually. Local erythema and swelling may occur and less often regional lymphadenopathy and pyrexia. In the UK this vaccine is prepared for the Department of Health and Social Security, Russell Square London by the Public Health Laboratory Service.

Botulism has not been reported as a laboratory infection but the vaccine is given when work with the toxin of Clostridium botulinum is done. A pentavalent toxoid aluminium phosphate-adsorbed vaccine is available from the Centers for Disease Control (CDC), Atlanta Georgia, USA. It contains toxoids from formalin-inactivated partially purified types A,B,C,D and E containing thiomersal as a preservative. The vaccine is given deep subcutaneously in a dose in a dose of 0.5 ml in three doses at intervals of 2 and 12 weeks with a booster dose at 12 months. Subsequent booster doses are required every 2 years but are only given if antibody levels judged by antitoxin levels in the serum are not satisfactory. Levels judged by antitoxin levels in the serum are not s satisfactory . At the time of writing Botulinum toxoid is not a licensed product in the USA and is only available under strict conditions laid down by CDC. Moderate local reactions do occur and are an indication to reduce subsequent doses.

The animal house

The general recommendations concerning staff health working in laboratories also apply in the specialised area of animal house. Conditions may be warm and dusty and the physical effort greater than in the main laboratory. Pulmonary diseases, especially of an allergic nature preclude employment there. Vaccinations against tuberculosis, rabies and tetanus are essential but other modes of protection of the animal attendant are equally important. These include the training of the worker so that he or she has some knowledge and understanding of animals, and that safe methods of handling and the means to do this are clear, Protective clothing clean clothing. And facilities for changing and showering are all important.

Animals are a reservoir of disease agents some of which can transmitted to man, and in some surveys have been shown to be the cause of over 10% of laboratory infection. Although the skin is often breached due to bites and scratches accidents with syringes and needles of ten occur in association with animals due to careless handling. Animals too are responsible for aerosols either from their fur or via urine and faeces allowed to dry in bedding. Such aerosols may be inhaled by handlers causing respiratory distress due to allergy. Material from animals can also get on to the hands and clothes of workers and thus be transmitted to the eyes.

The organisms being injected into the animals are also a hazard at this stage. Air in syringes should not be expelled into the room but into a small pledge of cotton wool soaked in disinfectant. It is also just as important to disinfect the skin of the animal after the injection as before. This is because the agent injected is frequently present at the site of infection and often is released into the atmosphere in the form of an aerosol. After injection the agent may be excreted via the urine, the faeces and open lesions, and from the respiratory tract in coughs and sneezes. Changing the bedding just as in a hospital ward, increases the number of bacteria detectable in the air.

Care should be exercised with animals newly introduced into the animal house. The stress of travel and of new surroundings and handlers may play a part in an increase susceptibility to disease. Animals may themselves be suffering from diseases such as tuberculosis but may be exposed to such a disease from a human handler. This situation is a particular hazard in monkey colonies. These animals may also be a source of Shigella and Salmonella infections as well as parasites such as Strongyloides, Entamoeba and Giardia. Adequate quarantine facilities will deal with these infections and the out-break of Marburg disease which occurred in Marburg, Frankfurt and Belgrade in 1967 is a salutory reminder of what can occur if quarantine regulations are ignored. Infection with B virus should not occur if only seronegative animals are used and screening for this highly dangerous disease should be done during the quarantine period.

Smaller animals are known to carry Salmonella, Yersinia, Leptospirosis and lymphocytic choriomeningitis, and outbreaks of disease in man have all been traced back to the 4 animal house. Skin infection appearing in animal handlers may be the first intimation of widespread infection of animals, with Trichophyton and Microsporon fungi. Toxoplasma and Toxocara may be caught from dogs and cats.

We do not know the risk form tumour viruses and indeed it may not exist at all because of species specificity. Nevertheless, we cannot ignore the possibility of transmission to man and hence materials derived from such tumour should be handled with care.

Special situation

HIV infections in health care workers

There is considerable apprehension among health care workers with regard to the dangers of handling blood from patients who are antibody positive to immunodeficiency virus. Guidelines for handling this material are available and concentrate on good basic techniques. No vaccine is available. Exposure to possible infection in health care workers due to splashing, cuts or needle stick injury must have occurred on thousands of occasions, but evidence of transmission of infection based on seroconversion appears to be confined to 19 cases, all of whom appear to have had substantial exposure to infection. There have also been a number of large surveys in which those exposed to infection as a result of a recorded incident have been followed up without any seroconversion taking place. Thus it is clear that handling HIV positive material is hazardous, but the risk is small and probably less than that from handling hepatitis B positive material. Such hazards should be clearly explained to all laboratory workers.

Pregnancy

The effects of rubella in pregnant women are well documented and similarly the dangers of Cytomegalovirus infection are understood. Other viruses are suspect as causes of malformation in babies if the mother is infected in the early stages of pregnancy. Many such infection may not be teratogenic, but a number such as mumps are associated with abortion. Women who are hoping to become pregnant, and those who are pregnant should not be allowed to work in a virus department. The chance of infection occurring elsewhere in the laboratory and causing harm is very low, so it is usual to move such female employees to a different task. This change in occupation can often be provided in the media preparation department or possibly handling environmental specimens such as food and water. The baseline serum collected on joining should have been tested for the presence of rubella and CMV antibodies and vaccination offered against the former. Cytomegalovirus, although clearly a cause of congenital infection, sometimes with severe abnormality in the off spring, is much less common. Vaccination is rarely done for female laboratory staff unless work with the virus is part of the research programme.

Absence due to illness

Staff should be instructed to send a message to

the laboratory when they are unable to work due to illness. This should always be done on the morning of the first day of absence. If no message is received a colleague should visit to make certain that the absentee is not suffering from some illness associated with his work. Such a step is of paramount importance if the employee is known to live alone.

Disaster services

Although it is unlikely that accidents can be before seen and plans made to cope with the incident an attempt should be made. The advantage of thinking a head in this context is that the exploration of an imagined incident in the form of discussion with those likely to be involved will stimulate ideas. These ideas should be committed to paper in an incident or disaster file, and should be available to all in authority at all times. The file should commence with a statement of the action to be taken by the staff involved in order (a) to mitigate the effects of the accident on him or her and (b) to prevent others being involved. This section of the file should be circulated to all staff and in large establishments where research is done staff should sign to signify that they have read the contents. The subsequent immediate action to be taken will depend upon agent involved and the degree of contamination which has taken place. This may be decided by the most senior member of the staff present at the time, or may concern the physician if he is called.

Subsequent entries in the file may be

administrative in the sense that it may simply consist of a list of names and telephone numbers of those who must be informed. Such lists are extremely useful in an emergency.

Finally the outline procedure should be laid down for an inquiry to be held. This should always be done however trivial the accident may seem, for it establishes two principles;

1. No grade of staff is immune from an injury;
2. All procedures leading up to the accident are liable to investigation are modification to prevent a repetition

Such a routine approach to all incidents establishes the fact that inquiries are not designed for disciplinary reasons but as a process in preventive health. Should disciplinary action be indicated this should follow a separate investigation by the employer and the physician should avoid taking part unless required to give medical evidence. It is most important that the preliminary internal inquiry should be established as a routine so that all staff are not afraid to report incidents or to co-operate in all the investigation.

12 Safety Precautions in a Clinical Laboratory

Introduction

Clinical cytogenetics has advanced considerably over the past decade and is moving ever closer to the rapidly developing field of recombinant DNA technology. DNA laboratories are currently being integrated into some existing cytogenetics departments and the training of laboratory workers now includes both disciplines. The DNA work is normally allocated space and personnel of its own, though there may be some rotation of staff for training purposes. Thus, the safety procedures in this part of the laboratory will differ from and extend beyond those in the cytogenetics section. However, health and safety procedures for the recombinant DNA technologist merit more attention than is appropriate in this chapter on cytogenetics. We have therefore, confined our attentions to the pure diagnostic cytogenetics laboratory.

Specimens dealt with in a cytogenetic laboratory–The potential risks

It is hoped that clinics will make every possible effort to inform the laboratory of any risks that may be associated with the samples they send . This information should be made clear on the request form and the sample labelled with the appropriate hazard warning sticker so that the laboratory can process it in accordance with the regulations relating to the particular pathogen involved. In practice, however, it should not be assumed that in the absence of such warning a specimen is without risk.

Samples form the following patients constitute the highest risks that are likely to confront the cytogeneticist, and these should always be dealt with by experienced staff in accordance with the strictest precautions;

1. Intravenous drug abusers. These are in high risk groups for both HIV and HBsAg;
2. Homosexual and bisexual. e .At risk for HIV;
3. Haemophiliacs. At risk for HIV;
4. Persons who have returned from sub-Sahara Africa during the last 5 years. At risk for HIV;
5. Sexual partners and babies of the above. At risk for HIV;
6. Patients who are Australia antigen positive;
7. Down's syndrome patients who are institutionalized. At risk for HBsAg due to immunosuppression;
8. Other immunosuppressed patients. At risk for HBsAg;
9. Unscreened patients from renal units. At risk for HBsAg,

10. Patients with suspected infective diseases of the liver. At risk for HBsAg; and
11. Babies with diarrhoea and vomiting. May be due to virulent pathogen.

The pathological specimens dealt with by most cytogenetics laboratories include blood amniotic fluid abortus material chorionic villi skin biopsy and some post-mortem material mostly from babies. Some laboratories also process bone marrow buccal smears, tumours testicular biopsics spleen lymph nodes and pleural effusions. Specimens sent for chromosome investigation are all potentially infective since they are received unfixed. Not all tissues, however, carry the same degree of risk.

Blood

Blood is a major source of potential infection. It is a particularly efficient transmitter of many pathogens especially HBsAg and HIV. All blood specimens including separated blood should be handled with particular caution.

Bone marrow and leukaemic blood

Granulocytopenia due either to the leukaemia itself or as a result of cytotoxic therapy is the most important factor increasing the risk of infection to these patients. Fungal and bacterial infections are those most commonly observed. Furthermore, damaged to natural barriers from cytotoxic therapy and invasive procedures carried out to aid diagnosis and administer treatment can produce routes for infection. Immunological impairment also occurs due to the effects of drugs or disease.

Over half of the documented infection in patients with leukaemia are due to hospital-acquired organisms. Virus infections rarely occur in patients with neutropenia. Herpes simplex, disseminated herpes zoster, severe herpes virus pneumonia and cytomegalovirus infection are also a major problem in transplantation patients.

The leukaemic patient may be transfused with blood products. Although these are now screened for the presence of HIV, the risks presented by these patients as a result of transfusion should be regarded as similar to the situation for haemophiliacs.

Epstein-Barr Virus

The supernatant from an Epstein-Barr Virus (EBV) producing cell line B95—8 is utilized in B-cell malignancies and for transforming lumphoblastic cell lines. It is a tumour promoter. Filtration is required prior to use and this must be done under the strictest safety conditions. A class 1 safety cabinet must be used for all cultures which have been in contact with EBV.

Amniotic fluid

Some amniotic fluid specimens may be contaminated with maternal blood and these carry the same risks as blood specimens. It is important to remember that some specimens may not be obviously bloodstained, but after centrifugation will show a small amount of blood in the pellet. For this reason, uncentrifuged amniotic fluid should be treated as potentially bloodstained and the appropriate precautions taken. A part from this, there is little risk of infection from an uncontaminated amniotic fluid specimen.

Chorionic villus samples

CVS samples are nearly always contaminated with maternal blood. In addition there is a small risk that contaminants from the cervix and vagina may be present.

Abortus material and stillbirths

The main risks of infection from this type of specimen are due to contact with maternal blood and body fluids. In some cases, spontaneous abortions may have occurred as a result of infection in the fetus, which may in turn present a risk of infection to the laboratory worker. Examples of such infections are syphilis, toxoplasmosis cytomegalovirus, herpes simplex type II, rubella, rubeola. For this reason, all products of conception should be treated with particular caution.

Skin biopsy, testicular biopsy and post-mortem tissues

All of these tissues have been in contact with blood and other body fluids and are, therefore capable of transmitting many pathogens, especially if the patient has died of an infection. However, since most of these samples will have come from babies, such material is a comparatively minor risk in the cytogenetics laboratory.

Lymph nodes, effusions, tumours, thymus, spleen

Contact with any malignant tissues requires stringent handling procedures. The aetiology of most malignancies is as yet unknown. However the is isolation of human T-cell-lymphoma-leudaemia virus (HTLV) from patients with T-cell leukaemia, sezary cell leukaemia and mycosis fungoides is the most direct evidence of a possible viral causation of human leukaemia. It should be borne in mind that vectors of malignant diseases may be present, but as yet undiscovered, and extreme caution should be exercised when handling potentially malignant material.

Pleural effusions carry a high risk of tuberculosis and should be handled with extreme caution by experienced staff who have a positive Mantoux reaction.

Buccal smears

Unfixed buccal smears are potentially capable of transmitting infections, especially when these cells have been in contact with infected sputum, but are of comparatively minor risk. This is the only type of sample that can be transported to the cytogenetics laboratory already fixed and clinics should be provided with the appropriate fixative for this purpose.

The collection, packaging and transport of specimens

The collection of specimens for chromosome analysis normally performed by clinicians, nursing staff or phlebotomists, on whom the cytogeneticist relies to take reasonable precautions to protect himself from the risk of infection from the sample. It is therefore, advisable that the laboratory should supply clinics and wards dealing with cytogenetics specimens with a concise protocol which be regularly updated and shown to new members of staff. It would be advantageous, where possible to encourage clinics to follow the procedure by supplying them with suitable containers plastic bags and boxes which should will help them to remember to use these items. When devising a protocol, the following points should be considered.

Containers

The use of plastic containers instead of glass for fluid specimens eliminates one of the most dangerous situations: that of broken glass contaminated with potentially infective material. Virtually all pathogens can be introduced through a wound. Most laboratories have now adopted the use of plastic containers.

Specimen containers should be leak-proof, easy to open and close securely without danger of infectioning the operator. Snap-on plug closures should be avoided as these produce a fine spray when opened. It is important to use containers which have a cap that does not trap part of the specimen between itself and the wall of the container. If a screw-cap is used, the thread should be on the outside of the neck of the container.

There are several designs of heparinized tube commercially available for the collection of blood samples suitable for cytogenetics. We would recommend the use of plastic screw-caped vessels and the avoidance of glass tubes with rubber bungs or snap-on plugs. Standard plastic screw-capped Universal containers are adequate for most other fluid samples. It is a good idea to seal the rim of these containers with parafilm if the sample is to be transported any distance.

Many cytogenetics laboratories receive entire fetuses from late abortions. These are best transported in the sweet 'jar' type of container or in a plastic bucket-style container.

Packaging

1. All containers should be transported in a sealed, sealed leak-proof bag; this is of particular importance when the specimen is fluid. Any leakage while in transit will be contained, there-by preventing potentially infective material form penetrating the outer packaging and exposing non-laboratory staff to the risk of infection.
2. When two or more specimens are to be sent in the same box, they should be sealed in separate plastic bags to prevent any cross-contamination.
3. Specimens in plastic bags should be packed in a strong box and padded tightly with absorbent material such as cellulose wadding or absorbent cotton wool. The box should be securely fastened, and preferably wrapped in a stout envelope or padded bag.
4. Hazard warning labels must be used where appropriate.

Request forms

Clinical staff should be asked to fill in request forms either before taking the specimen or after washing their hands having already taken the sample. This avoids contamination of request forms with potentially infective material. Similarly specimen containers should not be handled when a sample is being taken. If possible the labelling of containers and completing of request forms should be done before hand or by a colleague.

Request forms should never be put into the plastic bag with the specimen, or stapled to it, as these will become contaminated if the specimen should leak. Plastic bags designed to hold the form in a separate compartment are available commercially and these could be supplied to clinics with the containers and forms.

Clinics must always be informed immediately if a specimen arrives wrongly or badly packaged and every effort should be made to correct the mistakes of those people who habitually send material in this way.

Reception of specimens

A specimen which has been collected, packaged and transported properly should pose few problems for the recipient. The only precautions necessary in this case would be the receipt of the specimens by a trained person in a specifically allocated area of the laboratory. Specimen containers must only be opened in the appropriate safety cabinet. The following points should be considered when a specimen is received in a potentially dangerous condition.

Leakages

Laboratory coats and protective surgical gloves must always be worn when dealing with contaminated items.

Leakage contained in a plastic bag

It is a good idea to have a stock of disposable trays or similar receptacles on which leaking plastic bags and boxes can be placed inside the safety cabinet. If the entire specimen has leaked out be the container, the whole bag should be disposed of. If, however, some of the specimen has remained in the container and can be salvaged, it can be transferred into a fresh container. This is best achieved by getting a colleague to hold a new container ready so that when the leaking container is opened the remainder of the specimen can be transferred into the new container with a syringe or pipette. This avoids contamination of the new container. The bag container, tray and gloves can then be disposed of.

Leakage not contained in plastic bag

If potentially infective material has penetrated the outer packaging, all persons likely to have been in contact with the package must be informed immediately. The sender must also be notified as soon as possible. The package should be placed on a disposable tray, opened inside the safety cabinet and treated as for a contained leakage.

Leaking involving broken glass

The glass must not be touched once the package has been opened, but disposed of in the appropriate hazardous waste container.

Specimen container contaminated with specimen

The container should be treated as for 'contained' leak and the specimen transferred to a fresh container. The old container should be disposed of safely.

Request form contaminated with specimen

Details should be copied out into a fresh form, and the old form discarded in the appropriate hazardous waste container.

Processing the specimens

The principal ways in which unfixed pathological material can be brought into contact with the skin or mucous membranes are by:

1. The formation of aerosols and droplets;
2. Spillage and splashing;
3. Accidents involving sharp objects which may themselves be contaminated with the specimen, or which cause wounds through which pathogens may enter the body.

Safety precautions relating to the handling of pathological material are, therefore, designed to minimize the occurrence of such situations. They should also serve to provide adequate protection to the laboratory worker should such situations occur.

Most of the procedures used to prepare a specimen for chromosome analysis involve centrifugation, removal and replacement of supernatant and other reagents, resuspension of cell pellets, mixing and then fixation, after which the specimen ceases to be an infection risk.

General precautions

1. All unfixed material must be dealt with in a microbiological safety cabinet using full aseptic technique.

   Most specimens received in the cytogenetic laboratory can be handled in a class 2 cabinet. However, for some higher risk specimens such as HIV or HB_sAg a Class 1 cabinet should be used. High risk material should not be dealt with by a laboratory that does not possess, or have access to, the appropriate safety cabinet.

2. Laboratory coats and protective surgical gloves should be worn when dealing with all unfixed pathological materials.

3. The hands must never be brought into contact with the eyes, nose or mouth during the handling of any biological material.

4. If it is necessary to answer the telephone or attend to other such matters during the processing of a specimen, the gloves should be first removed and discarded. A fresh pair of gloves should be put on when processing is resumed.

5. Plastic containers, culture vessels and other utensils should be used in preference to glass, to avoid accidents involving infected broken glass.

6. Care must be taken to ensure that the tips of dispensers, wash bottles etc., are not brought into contact with the unfixed specimen or contaminated containers when adding reagents to cultures.

7. Syringes should be used without needles where possible. An example of this is the aliquoting of a blood sample from a heparinized tube to a culture vessel.

8. Replacing a contaminated needle in a sheath is extremely dangerous if done hastily. It is preferable to remove the needle from the syringe and discard it in a 'sharps' bin. If the sheath must be replaced, this should be done very carefully.

9. Centrifugation should be carried out in plastic tubes which are securely stoppered. Sealed buckets should be used, if possible, since these are more efficient than sealed rotors. The buckets should be opened in the safety cabinet if unfixed material has been centrifuged.

10. Operations requiring mechanical blending should be done in tightly stoppered tubes. Even mixing by hand requires tightly stoppered tubes.

11. Pouring liquid cultures and supernatants should be discouraged even if carried out in a safety cabinet. Spillage is likely to occur from time to time, especially if the operator is an inexperienced trainee.

12. If suction pumps, etc. are used for removal of supernatant, the expelled air must be filtered and exhausted with the outflow from the cabinet. Most safety cabinets are designed to facilitate the incorporation of an outflow pipe from a pump into the exhaust system.

Incubation

Cultures which are grown in an 'open' system require that the caps of the vessel be loosened by a turn of the thread. Overfilling of these vessels should be avoided since leakage of contaminated medium can easily occur. Some designs of Leighton on tube are especially prone to this, particularly if they roll over when accidentally knocked. It is good practice to stack culture vessels in racks or on trays which can be removed from the incubator and decontaminated. This prevents contamination of incubator shelves should leakage occur.

Some cytogenetic procedures require the addition of hazardous reagents during the incubation period. These are discussed in detail in a later section.

Disposal of contaminated waste

Every hospital or institution dealing with pathological material will have strict regulations regarding the disposal of infected or potentially infected waste, and every laboratory worker must be familiar with these procedures. The decontamination of waste pathological material is dealt with extensively, and information applicable to the cytogenetic laboratory. We will not, therefore, reiterate this at great length. However, to summarize briefly:

Hypodermic syringes and scalpel blades

'Sharps' and broken glass can normally be placed in commercially available boxes or containers with imperforate, not readily penetrable, walls which can be autoclaved and incinerated.

Discarded specimens, cultures, contaminated disposables

These should be placed in metal or heat-resistant plastic containers and autoclaved before leaving the laboratory. They should then be incinerated. Large volumes of fluid may be emptied into a sink or sluice connected to the public sewer, or treated with a disinfectant such as hypochlorite or glutaraldehyde. If solid tissue is disinfected overnight it should be poured through a sieve over the sink so that the liquid can be washed down and the solid tissue autoclaved and incinerated.

Disinfectants

Clear phenolics should be used for most organic matter other than blood. This is suitable for disinfecting metal instruments after setting up tissues for culturing, since phenolics do not attack metal. Hypochlorite should be used for blood including those which may be at risk for HBsAg, but should never be used for equipment with metal parts since hypochlorites attack metal.

Safely precautions to be taken when handling chemicals and reagents

All chemicals and reagents used in the cytogenetic laboratory must be handled with caution, even if there is no particular known risk associated with a specific substance. Protective clothing and gloves should be worn whenever chemicals are to be handled. Before dealing with the different chemicals commonly used in cytogenetic laboratory, it is necessary to draw attention to the following general safety precautions.

1. Mouth pipetting of all chemicals, reagents and specimens should be strictly forbidden.
2. All chemicals and reagents should be clearly labelled and bear the relevant international standard hazard warning symbols.
3. Both hands should be used when carrying large bottles containing chemicals and reagents one hand being used to support the bottle from its base.
4. Large bottles of chemicals should be transported in carriers specifically designed for this purpose, with one hand free to give support.
5. When solutions are prepared in large flasks the flask, should not be held by the neck and rotated since breakage could easily occur.
6. Chemical solutions should never be poured from a container being held above eye level. The recipient container should be held firmly on the bench while the solution is being gently poured into it.

Corrosive chemicals–acids and alkalis

Corrosive fluids should be stored on low shelves, or preferably in an 'inflammables' store if this is appropriate. Bottles containing strong acids should be opened with extreme caution, in a fume cupboard. Protective safety spectacles should also be worn while dealing with these corrosive substances. Since an exothermic reaction occurs when water is added to strong acids, dilutions must only be produced by adding measured amounts of the acid to the water slowly, mixing them until the desired amount of acid has been added. Acids and alkalis can be disposed of down the sink as long as they are thoroughly diluted and the water is run for a few minutes afterwards.

The following corrosive chemicals are those commonly used in cytogenetics:

Glacial acetic acid

Acetic acid is in constant use in the cytogenetic laboratory since it is mixed with methanol (1:3) to make the fixative used for processing all samples. Although considered a weak acid acetic acid in glacial form is highly corrosive. This acid, must always be handled in a fume cupboard since harmful vapours are produced and it must be kept away from heat, naked flames and sparks.

Hydrochloric acid

Concentrated HCl may be used with 70% ethanol for the cleaning of cover slips or slides which are used for culturing. but 0.d2 N HCI is the strength more commonly used for C-banding. If a laboratory uses this acid in both strengths it is a good idea to but the 0.2 N strength commercially rather than prepare the dilution form concentrate thus minimizing the need for handling the more dangerous concentrate. Concentrated HCI is corrosive, poisonous and produces a harmful vapour which readily destroys the mucous membranes, producing violent irritation of the upper respiratory tract.

Sodium hydroxide/potassium/barium hydroxide

These are extremely corrosive substances. Barium hydroxide is particularly toxic. This is used in C-banding and care should be taken when weighing out this substance.

Inflammable chemicals

Alcohols and solvents may be toxic as well as inflammable. All highly inflammable chemicals must be stored in a metal cabinet with a secure lock at a suitable level such that access is not impaired. This cabinet must be clearly marked with the appropriate hazard warning label. These chemicals should be handled within fume cupboard.

Large stocks of solvents must be kept outside the laboratory in a cool fire-proof store, and when they are brought in from such a cool store, the stopper must be loosened cautiously. Any solvent stocks to be stored within the laboratory must be stored in metal containers in a cool place.

Since solvent vapors can travel a long way they may cause 'flashback' from a distant Bunsen burner. All burners must, therefore, be extinguished prior to the use of a solvent, or be kept in a separate room.

Care should be taken in the collection of solvents to avoid incompatible reactions; indeed, some substances can be explosive under certain conditions. Solvents and alcohols should never be poured down the sink since to do this constitutes a fire hazard and some local authorities forbid their disposal into the main drainage systems. Inflammable waste should be collected into metal drums which should be stored in a cool place until their periodic disposal by a professional firm.

The following inflammable chemicals are those in common use in the cytogenetic laboratory:

Methanol

Methanol is the most commonly used alcohol in the cytogenetic laboratory since the fixative made by adding it to glacial acetic acid is used for the processing of cultures. It is often used for destaining slides. Methanol is highly inflammable, and toxic both by ingestion and inhalation:

Ethanol

Ethanol is the other commonly used alcohol both in absolute concentration, and 70% dilution. This like all alcohols is highly inflammable. Excessive inhalation may produce intoxication and tolerance.

Fixative

The 3:1 methanol: acetic fixative is used daily in cytogenetic laboratories. Like all fixatives it is poisonous chemical solution which causes coagulation of the proteins which make tissues firm and solid, thus preventing natural liquefaction. Living skin may also be fixed if in contact with fixative for 15 minutes or more. Gloves should therefore, always be worn when working with this fixative, and procedures carried out in a fume cupboard.

Xylene

Xylene is the most common solvent found in the

cytogenetic laboratory as it is the component of many slide mountants such as DPX. It may also be used for cleaning microscope slides. Aromatic hydrocarbon solvents such as xylene are volatile and toxic by all portals of entry and should, therefore always be dealt with in a fume cupboard. Xylene fumes may build up during a session of slide mounting so this should be done in a well ventilated area or within a fume cupboard.

Toxic, cytotoxic and carcinogenic chemicals and reagents

An increasing number of toxic, cytotoxic and potentially carcinogenic chemicals are being used in cytogenetic laboratory as techniques become more sophisticated. In addition to the precautions already outlined above, it is advisable to wear an effective face mask whenever this category of reagent is used. This prevents inhalation of dust from the powdered forms, and particular care should be taken when using balances to weigh out these chemicals.

Aerosol formation from solutions of these reagents is as dangerous to the operator as aerosols from high-risk samples. These chemicals should never be handled on the open bench.

Material should be reduced to a non-carcinogenic state prior to disposal into a sewer or waste collection system. For instance, quinacrine mustard should be treated with hypochlorite solution. Controls for the use of carcinogens in hospitals are very strict, and staff should be familiar with their local code of conduct. Only experienced workers should handle such reagents.

Many of the chemicals and reagents used in the cytogenetic laboratory are harmful on ingestion or inhalation, or are irritants. Care should be taken not to introduce them into the mouth by nail-biting, sucking of fingers, etc. other reagents which should be handled with caution include: Distamycin A, DAPI, Hoechst 33258, deoxycytidine, phytohaemagglutinin, pokeweed mitogen, DMSO, copper sulphate, silver nitrate immersion oil, hydrogen peroxide.

Antibiotics and fungicides

The use of antibiotics and fungicides should be restricted to a minimum since resistant strains of pathogenic organisms can be established in the laboratory environment by excessive use. Those commonly used in the cytogenetic laboratory are penicillin streptomycin, gentamicin polymyxin, mycostatin, amphoteracin B.

Enzymes

Trypsin is commonly used in the cytogenetic laboratory. Collagenase may be used for some tissue cultures. Enzymes may cause allergic reactions in some people and gloves should be worn for handling.

It should be remembered that even the most innocuous reagents such as salts amino acids and enzymes may be harmful if ingested and care should be taken even when dealing with these. Absence of a warning sign should not be regarded as a guarantee of safety. If any substance is new or unfamiliar and the hazards are not displayed on the items safety data sheets should be made available from the custom services departments of the companies supplying these reagents.

Compressed and liquefied gases

CO_2 Gas cylinders

These are used to produce a 0.5% CO_2 level inside incubators used for tissue culture. These cylinders should be placed outside the premises and protected from extremes of temperature. Warning notices should be displayed where the cylinders are stored and used and trolleys should always be used to transport them. They must be securely supported during use and placed in a position such that they can be easily removed in an emergency. Water should always be used when testing valve sockets for leakages.

When operating the cylinder the valve should be opened slowly at first and then no more than is necessary to obtain the gas flow required. Cylinder valves gauge regulators or other fittings must not be oiled or greased at any time and white lead or paint must never be applied to them.

Liquid nitrogen

This is used in equipment for the freezing and storage of cells. It is important that proper protective clothing should be worn when handling liquid nitrogen, this consisting of a laboratory coat, asbestos gloves with long arms and a transparent face shield. Sandals or open shoes should not be worn in case of splashes to the feet. The room must be well ventilated when pouring liquefied gases and they must not be poured near flames. Metal objects which have been immersed in liquid nitrogen must not be touched with the bare hands since they can cause severe burns to the skin. Care should betaken over the storage of ampoules in liquid nitrogen. If nitrogen is trapped in a badly sealed ampoule, the ampoule will explode when it is withdrawn. Surrounding the ampoule with cotton wool or cloth will lessen the risk.

Safety precautions to be taken with equipment

centrifuges

Precautions relating to the treatment of specimens to be centrifuged and the action to be taken in case of accidents involving specimens in the centrifuge have already been discussed. The following safety measures are therefore concerned solely with the prevention of risk room use of the machine itself.

The entire centrifuge and accessories should be cleaned regularly and the bowl, head and accessories should be disinfected. All items should be autoclaved where possible. Centrifuges can be very dangerous if not operated correctly and must be properly maintained and serviced at regular intervals. Only the heads and accessories recommended by the manufacturer must be used as replacement parts. Because corrosion is the main cause of centrifuge failure, all heads and accessories should be inspected frequently for signs of corrosion and hair cracks. Accessories and contents must be carefully balanced and the load distributed symmetrically around the head before starting the centrifuge. The containers must be of a size correct for the swing-out heads to ensure that there is an adequate clearance when the horizontal position is reached.

All centrifuges used in the cytogenetic laboratory must have sealed buckets and there must be a few minutes pause after the rotor has come to rest during which the lid cannot be opened. The centrifuges should be of a type which will not operate unless the lid is securely fastened. The centrifuge must never be stopped by turning it off at the mains neither should the head be stopped by hand. All changes in speed must be made slowly.

Microscopes

These should be properly adjusted and cleaned regularly to minimize straining the eyes. Good quality microscopes should be used for the analysis of banded preparations since this in particular can cause severe eyestrain if an unsuitable microscope is continually used. It is advisable to site microscopes to be used for banding analysis in a room with daylight and a fairly long-distance view so that the eyes can be relaxed on this periodically during long session of such analysis.

CO_2 Incubators

These should not be situated in a small room unless there is an adequate ventilation system since the CO_2 level in the atmosphere may reach too high a level. Care should be taken to avoid condensation from humidified incubators reaching electrical components of machine. Incubators should be cleaned at least it once a week with non-hypochlorite disinfectant. All spillage of pathological material must be cleaned with swabs and cotton wool and non-hypochlorite disinfectant.

Cell banks

Cell banks containing liquid nitrogen must not situated in a small sealed room unless there is adequate ventilation since the level of nitrogen may build up and cause suffocation.

Water baths

These should not be used at temperatures in excess of 80°C. Some R-banding methods necessitate the use of water baths at 88°C for about '10 minutes, if this is to be done the work should be carried out as quickly and carefully as possible and the temperature of the water reduced as soon as this treatment has been completed. This should however be avoided if possible since the danger of scalding is considerable.

Index